Susan Clark was voted Health Journalist of the Year in 2000 and was the first health and fitness editor for the *Sunday Times*, where her hugely popular 'What's the Alternative?' column appears each week. She is a regular contributor to many national magazines, journals and newspapers and, as an experienced broadcaster, attracts massive audiences on both radio and television. She also acts as a consultant to several herbal companies and the Health Food Manufacturers' Association and is a British Wheel of Yoga-trained teacher. She lives in Oxfordshire with her husband and young daughter.

Also by Susan Clark

WHAT REALLY WORKS
The Insider's Guide to Natural Health
What's Best and Where to Find it

THE VITALITY COOKBOOK

WHAT REALLY WORKS FOR KIDS

The Insider's Guide to Natural Health for Mums and Dads

SUSAN CLARK

BANTAM PRESS

LONDON · NEW YORK · TORONTO · SYDNEY · AUCKLAND

TRANSWORLD PUBLISHERS
61–63 Uxbridge Road, London W5 5SA
a division of The Random House Group Ltd

RANDOM HOUSE AUSTRALIA (PTY) LTD
20 Alfred Street, Milsons Point, Sydney,
New South Wales 2061, Australia

RANDOM HOUSE NEW ZEALAND LTD
18 Poland Road, Glenfield, Auckland 10, New Zealand

RANDOM HOUSE SOUTH AFRICA (PTY) LTD
Endulini, 5a Jubilee Road, Parktown 2193, South Africa

Published 2002 by Bantam Press
a division of Transworld Publishers

A catalogue record for this book is available from the British Library.
ISBN 0593 049195

Note: all prices were correct at the time of going to press.

The publisher has used its best endeavours to ensure that the URLs for external websites referred
to in this book are correct and active at the time of going to press. However, the publisher has no
responsibility for the websites and can make no guarantee that a site will remain live or that the
content is or will remain appropriate.

Typeset in Sabon by Falcon Oast Graphic Art Ltd

Printed in Great Britain by
Mackays of Chatham, Chatham, Kent

1 3 5 7 9 10 8 6 4 2

For my sister, Melissa

Note

The health advice in this book is intended to guide parents to make healthier choices for their children. It is not to be treated as a substitute for medical advice from your family doctor or any other qualified medical practitioner. This is important because natural medicines, such as herbs, can be every bit as powerful as prescription drugs (which is, of course, why they work) and are likely to interact with existing medication. Doctors who are sympathetic to complementary medicine are better able to advise on the likelihood and the consequences of such interactions.

Contents

PART FIVE

An A–Z Guide to Natural Remedies for Everyday Complaints

Acknowledgements

With grateful thanks to Declan O'Mahony, Chelsea, the Goose Club and Harriet Griffey, who all know why. Special thanks to my agent, Teresa Chris, and my editor, Brenda Kimber at Transworld.

Come to the edge, he said.
They said: 'We are afraid.'
Come to the edge, he said.
They came.
He pushed them . . . and they flew.

Guillaume Apollinaire

Preface

Physicians treat but nature heals

What is the single greatest gift you can give your child? Vibrant good health, of course. But in a world where children as young as ten are being diagnosed with early signs of heart disease, where computers, not dogs, are a child's best friend, and where up to a third of the young children in an infant school may be taking Ritalin – a drug with a toxicology similar to that of cocaine – how do you get it right?

According to the World Health Organization (WHO) – the health monitoring arm of the United Nations – some 80 per cent of the world's population still relies on natural healing as their primary form of healthcare. Modern pharmacology has its very roots in herbal medicine and if you need a place to start practising a more holistic approach to life, there is none better than the next generation.

Children's bodies are wonderfully responsive to natural medicine. Children know instinctively how to get better, and what they need from you is nurture, support and care to guide them through. Sick children sleep a lot, eat very little, run a fever to kill off bugs and use their energy to kick-start the body's own healing processes. What you can do – using *What Really Works for Kids* – is give nature a nudge. For example, instead of treating a cold with an over-the-counter remedy that suppresses the symptoms, why not use a herb like echinacea that can support the immune system instead? Remember, the first doctors were shamans and the first medicines were plants.

Natural medicine is gentle, effective and, when you know what you are doing, 100 per cent safe. As well as guiding confused and often scared parents through the maze of political hot-potato issues that surround child health, such as vaccination and hyperactivity, *What Really Works for Kids* tells you how your child's body changes over the years and what you can do to support those changes.

You will learn how to interpret deliberately confusing food and vitamin labels to screen out toxic chemicals and artificial sweeteners, and how to treat childhood illnesses in ways that support and strengthen the body's own natural processes. You'll even become a whizz at hiding remedies in everyday foods and in making smoothies and substitute meals that are bursting with vitality for faddy eaters and stroppy teens.

You'll find out how you can practise yoga with your child or children so that they keep their natural strength and flexibility, and how to discreetly control food portions to discourage overeating and obesity – a condition that now affects one in three children by the age of eleven.

This is not an either/or approach. If you want to take your kids to the doctor – and if they have an acute condition you must take them – that's fine. What we then do is show you how to support your children's system if they are given prescription drugs, and how to 'clear up' and detox a body after sickness.

Nobody told me how hard being a parent was going to be – how tiring, how thankless (some of the time) and how scary. This is not just a book for kids, it's also for you, Mum and Dad, and so there are also lots of tips on things you can do and use to keep yourself fighting fit enough to survive and even enjoy their childhood.

This is *the guide* for parents who want to build better and lasting health for their children, and for anyone who knows that, when it comes to kids, nature and the kids' own growing bodies have most of the answers.

PART ONE

Health Hazards,
Traps and Traumas

Introduction

Open any newspaper, any day of the week, and you will quickly realize how tough it is to be a parent and to protect your kids from all the health hazards and pitfalls that have become a fact of their everyday lives, whether it's a report of gender-bending chemicals in typical 'kid' foods such as baked beans, or yet another story linking (or dismissing any link between) the measles, mumps and rubella (MMR) triple-dose vaccine and frightening conditions such as autism or Crohn's disease. You'll find stories about headteachers sending letters home to parents warning them that their child – like one in three children in this country now – is dangerously overweight, and stories about junk-food diets making kids' brains, as well as their waistlines, flabbier.

You'll try to switch to an organic diet where possible and then you'll read yet another government report telling you you're wasting your money because nobody has really shown any significant difference in nutritional value between organic and non-organic produce. (They're not worried about the residues of pesticides and other agricultural chemicals used in the production of foods from nutritionally depleted soils then?) And nobody's going to tell you that a large number of the so-called 'health' supplements and drinks on sale contain additives, especially artificial sweeteners, which many researchers believe to be carcinogenic. It's going to be hard to cut out all additives – unless you move to a yoga ashram – so the best way to protect your family is to find out which are the ones you need to worry about most, to start reading the food labels that the manufacturers don't want you to understand anyway, and to avoid buying foods that contain the worst offenders. This section shows you how easy it is to start doing just that.

The fact is, however careful you are or well informed you try to be, it has never been more difficult to keep your kids healthy or to sort fact from fiction. That is why this important section starts the book. In it, you'll learn why some parents don't want to comply with the government's vaccination programme and what your alternatives are if you decide to opt out too. Even if you have had your children vaccinated, you'll learn how you can use complementary medicine to then support the immune system and restore optimum health.

If your family is struggling to cope with a child who has been diagnosed as suffering from Attention Deficit Disorder (ADD) or Attention Deficit Hyperactivity Disorder (ADHD), you will find out why neuroscientists and nutritionists believe supplementing the diet with essential fatty acids (EFAs) and zinc holds the key. If your child is depressed – and one in ten kids aged five to fifteen are – you will learn about your alternatives to giving them antidepressant drugs that were originally formulated for adults.

Maybe you have a high-achieving child who's suddenly been felled by chronic fatigue. Did you know there's a humble UK hedgerow berry which can not only rebuild a battered immune system but also works specifically against the Epstein-Barr virus

(EBV) many researchers now believe plays a key role in this debilitating disease?

This is the section that will also show you how to recognize and cope with the symptoms of a disease that is every parent's nightmare – meningitis – and how to help an obese child stay motivated to change his or her diet and not only lose weight but keep that weight off for good. How? By using an extraordinary substance that scientists found not in raw salads or healthy fruits but in that staple of kids' junk fare – the flame-grilled hamburger.

Intrigued?

Read on.

The Vaccine Debate

When you have to decide whether to follow the 'herd' and vaccinate your child or whether to resist, it can feel as if you're damned if you do and damned if you don't. This is one of the toughest decisions parents must face, not least because none of the so-called experts can agree on whether there really is any need to worry about a link to reported and alarming side effects such as autism and Crohn's disease. First, one set of scientists publishes a report saying the link between the triple MMR vaccine and a risk of your child developing autism is very real. Then another, equally reputable group of researchers publishes its results, saying rubbish, it's all a load of hot air. Stuck in the middle, like a ping-pong ball (and given about as much consideration), are the poor parents who are only trying to do what is right and what is best for their children and their long-term health.

What to do

Make an **informed choice**. Your health visitor and doctor will bombard you with information about the dangers of not vaccinating your child. Just to make sure you feel really scared, you'll even see over-the-top government TV ads showing wild cats prowling towards an abandoned and defenceless baby, implying, of course, you will be acting just as irresponsibly as this child's parent if you don't vaccinate. But don't fall at the first fence and don't let yourself be bullied.

If you've not yet decided what to do, read the recommended books on page 10 and talk to the support groups on page 12 before deciding whether to (a) go ahead, (b) seek an alternative or (c) go ahead and then use complementary medicine to support your child's immune system through the vaccination programme. Those are three of your options. Your remaining option is to go ahead with the vaccinations but to find a practitioner who will administer single-dose vaccines instead of the triple dose of the MMR. The theory behind this as an alternative route is that in nature your child would never be bombarded with measles, mumps and rubella all at once, and that to assault a child's immature immune system with all three vaccines at the same time will only confuse and weaken it (see page 268 for more on how the immune system and thus vaccination actually works).

Your starting point, before you make any decision, is to find out how vaccines work and which ones your child will be expected to have and when.

The UK Vaccination Schedule
(Or when you'll be expected to make sure they get their jabs)

In America and France, kids cannot access school unless their vaccination programme is up to date. Here in the UK, the recommended immunization schedule (see below) remains voluntary. That said, you will feel under pressure to comply, and if you do, with the addition of the relatively new and genetically modified meningitis C vaccine, your child will now get a total of twenty-one shots of infectious agents before the age of two.

2 months: vaccination against polio, HIB,* diphtheria, tetanus, meningitis C and whooping cough

3 months: second vaccination against polio, HIB, diphtheria, tetanus, meningitis C and whooping cough

4 months: third vaccination against polio, HIB, diphtheria, tetanus, meningitis C and whooping cough

12–15 months: first MMR (against measles, mumps and rubella)

3–5 years: pre-school MMR booster, plus diphtheria, tetanus and polio (DTP)

10–13 years: tuberculosis (BCG), although this is sometimes given soon after birth

14–19 years: diphtheria, tetanus booster and polio

*HIB stands for Haemophilus Influenza type B; a bacterial strain of meningitis which is most harmful to babies and kids under four. In one person per 1,000, a weakened immune system will allow this bacterium to pass into the brain, causing HIB.

How These Vaccines Work

There are three ways in which vaccines are made to confer active immunity on your child.

1) With the **MMR,** the micro-organisms that cause these diseases are injected in a live but weakened (or attenuated) form to trigger the immune system to make the antibodies (see Immune System, page 268) to destroy them. What happens then, when your child is exposed for real, is that the immune system, which can remember previous infections and has learned how to eradicate them, is already geared up to wipe the organisms out. It is because the organisms in this vaccine are still live that your child may suffer a mild form of measles or some other inflammatory response some ten days or so after the vaccination.

2) The **whooping cough** vaccine works by injecting dead organisms which have the 'shape' of the invading organism – which is known as the antigen (or pathogen) – but which cannot divide or multiply in the body. Again, the immune system's fighting forces (white blood cells and other proteins) recognize these as foreign invaders and make a memory of the shape for future attacks.

3) With both the **tetanus** and **diphtheria** vaccines, toxoids made from the bacteria's own toxins (but which have been modified and made non-toxic) are injected. Although no longer toxic, they still trigger the immune system to form antibodies that will destroy them and the real thing during any subsequent exposure.

Reported side effects and who's saying what?

- Children very rarely die of the side effects of vaccination; far more common are a range of symptoms including thrush, recurrent ear infections, insomnia, aggressive behaviour, allergies, an inability to concentrate, eczema, and other health problems parents (and kids) simply learn to put up with.
- The whooping-cough vaccination has been controversially linked with neurological problems in some patients.
- Research work has also shown that, in some autistic children, there are large amounts of the measles virus in the lymph glands and in the intestines, presumably from vaccination.
- Parents are also concerned about the use of mercury – a substance your dentist must treat as toxic waste outside of your mouth – as a preservative in DTP, the vaccines designed to protect against diphtheria, tetanus and polio. This highlights a general problem with all vaccines which are laced with other substances designed to disinfect, enhance their action or bind the component parts together.

MMR – The Autism Connection

The research that first suggested a link between the MMR jab and autism was carried out by Dr Andrew Wakeman, a gastro-enterologist formerly at the Royal Free Hospital in London. His findings were subsequently rubbished by other researchers who claim that, despite using even more sensitive techniques, they cannot be replicated. This has done nothing to allay parental fears and, at the time of going to press, around five hundred families are involved in preparing a legal claim for compensation.

Interestingly, those who dismissed Dr Wakeman's findings may yet find themselves eating humble pie since newer research carried out at the Royal Free Hospital, which was based not on statistical analysis but on indisputable clinical findings, reports a high incidence of the condition leaky gut (see page 170) – which some experts believe may be a reaction to the MMR vaccine – in children diagnosed with autism. These findings are further supported by US research by child specialists at the University of Minnesota, Minneapolis, who reported that out of 35 autistic children, 27 were found to have abnormal immune systems, a defect that also plays a critical role in leaky gut.

Taking an Informed Step

If you have not completed the vaccination programme, first read:

- *Immunization – Everything You Need to Know About Vaccinations and Immune-Boosting Therapies for Your Child* by ex-paediatric staff nurse and widely respected children's health writer Harriet Griffey. Published by Element, it costs £7.99.

- *Vaccination – The Hidden Facts* and *Health – The Only Immunity (The Alternative to Vaccination)*, both written and published by Australian naturopath Ian Sinclair. To order either book, e-mail the author on surflower45@hotmail.com.

If you have already vaccinated and want to find out more about how to support your child's immune system now, read:

- *An Educated Decision: One Approach to the Vaccination Problem Using Homeopathy* by London-based homeopath Christina J. Head. Published by the Lavender Hill Publishing Company (020 7978 4519), it costs £9.99 plus £1 p&p.

The Alternatives

Homeopathy

Stephen Langley is an Australian-trained naturopath and father of two, who shunned the conventional route and instead successfully boosted his own children's immunity using homeopathic vaccinations. With a homeopathic vaccination, potencies of the various diseases, including measles, mumps and whooping cough, are given at the same key stages of development as regular vaccinations. (To find out how homeopathy works, see pages 114–18. To understand why it works in the same way as a vaccine to boost immunity, see the Immune System, pages 268–76.)

Stephen Langley practises at the Hale Clinic in London (020 7631 0156) and can be contacted by e-mail: info@holohealth.com.

Christina Head is another London-based and highly skilled homeopath and author who understands all the issues that parents facing the vaccination debate must unravel. She can report excellent results from her method of treating both children who have been vaccinated and those whose parents opted for an alternative route. Her very persuasive theory is that many of the everyday health niggles parents and kids simply learn to put up with – complaints such as constant runny noses, eczema, recurrent ear infections and asthma – are a legacy of vaccination. And she has shown how, once you use homeopathy to 'clear' what she calls the residual pattern or vibration of sickness left behind, you can restore the body to optimum health and get rid of these kinds of debilitating and often difficult-to-treat conditions.

Christina J. Head practises at the Lavender Hill Clinic (020 7978 4519). Her clinical results are published in her recommended book, see page 10.

Single-dose Vaccines

Although many agencies are adamant there is no proven link between the MMR vaccine and autism, or the whooping-cough vaccine and neurological problems, many parents would prefer their child to be vaccinated with single doses only. The trouble with this is that doctors who have been willing to provide single-dose vaccines, which they have to import from Europe, have run the risk of being struck off. (Some UK parents have travelled to France to circumvent this problem but how many families have the money to do that, at the right time, for every child?)

There is no evidence that single-dose vaccination is safer than the triple dose, but only because nobody has bothered yet to research the question. What the government will argue is that single-dose vaccines expose your child to more risk since you have to wait several weeks between jabs and during those waits your child is unprotected from the diseases they have not yet been vaccinated against. (For as long as herd immunity is maintained (see page 13), this argument is not going to sway many concerned parents, selfish or otherwise.)

If you are looking for a practitioner who is qualified to administer single-dose vaccines, contact Dr Peter Mansfield at Replete (formerly Good HealthKeeping) on 01507 601655. Any of the following support groups can also help you make a more independent decision:

- Vaccination Awareness Network 08704 440894
- What Doctors Don't Tell You 020 7354 4592
- JABS (Justice, Awareness and Basic Support) 01942 713565
- The Informed Parent 020 8861 1022

Herd Immunity

Childhood diseases such as measles and mumps are now almost unheard of in Britain, thanks to vaccination. But to keep these conditions stamped out, the immunity of a critical mass of the population – what is called 'herd' immunity – must be maintained. When this happens, the minority of children who have not been vaccinated are de facto protected.

In the case of measles, this critical mass is 95 per cent of the population. In reality now, the uptake on vaccination is down to 88 per cent, which is why you will hear some health professionals predicting a measles epidemic.

Remember, too, that the higher number of kids doctors vaccinate, the more money they earn. (Currently £910 a year for a 70 per cent take-up, rising to £2,730 if they hit a target of 90 per cent.) I am not implying anything improper here but when you are seeking neutral and independent advice, this may be one of the factors nobody bothers to mention, while they are busy making you feel like a criminal for daring to question the 'system'.

Quick-fix Treat

Energy Gel It sounds too good to be true but there really is a gel that can give you a much-needed energy boost. With pure extracts of immune-boosting echinacea, yarrow, horsetail, lemon balm and ginger, for best results use it after a refreshing shower. Said to work in conjunction with lymphatic drainage, it promises to clear energy blocks and rejuvenate tissues, leaving you full of beans and raring to go. Energy Gel costs £11.90 for a 30ml tube and is available from Higher Nature on 01435 882880. Massage into a tired body.

Obesity, Dieting and Eating Disorders

By the age of eleven, a third of all UK kids are obese. And it hasn't happened overnight. For most, the weight starts to pile on at the age of nine. I could spend the rest of this section listing and elaborating on all the reasons why we're now breeding a generation of heavy-weights – gameboys, computers, digital TV, remote controls, schools with no playgrounds, nobody walking to school any more and parents too scared to give kids the freedom to disappear for hours and run around with their pals – but I'd rather devote the space to telling you what, as parents, we can do about it and how to help your child maintain a healthy weight.

With kids as young as eight now being treated for eating disorders (see page 18), dieting is not the answer. In fact, since so many dieters, young and old, regain not only the weight they successfully lost but more, it never has been. The only way to achieve and then maintain an optimum weight is to move away from the typical high-fat, high-sugar, low-fibre diet that caused the problem in the first place, and move towards a healthier way of eating. (For more guidance on this shift, including recipes, see Part Three, Food Talk.) Explain to your child (especially to teen girls) that skipping meals and following starvation diets cannot work in the long term. When the body is starved it steps up the rate at which fat stores are laid down so it will have an adequate supply for the hard times ahead. In other words, you will get fatter.

The Good News . . .

The good news is that you and the kids can eat as much as you like . . . of the right kinds of foods. This means you won't go hungry. You can then save the wrong kinds of foods to have as an occasional treat. The worst thing you can do is ban certain foods altogether or make a huge issue out of what's wrong with junk foods. Researchers at the Department of Human Development and Family Studies at Pennsylvania University, for example, found that kids whose mothers banned unhealthy fizzy drinks and sweets were more likely to eat them in secret than kids whose parents had not clamped down.

The Even Better News . . .

To help you and your child stay within an optimum weight, you can use a dietary supplement that is so successful it became the top-selling supplement in South Africa just weeks after its launch there in the summer of 2000. Bizarrely, the amazing nutrient that can help to control weight is one that is found naturally in . . . wait for it . . . the flame-grilled hamburger! This doesn't mean you can book a season ticket to McDonald's because hamburgers are also packed with unhealthy saturated fats which will make the scales carry on tipping the wrong way. But the way that scientists found this substance, which is called **conjugated linoleic acid** and is always shortened to the name **CLA,** is a great tale.

Their brief was not to find a weight-management nutrient but to work out what happened to meat when you cook it and to assess how many cancer-causing substances (carcinogens) are generated when great slabs of meat are cooked at high temperatures on, say, the family barbecue or under the grill. The researchers found potential carcinogens, yes. Especially when the meat was charred on the outside. But what they also found was a mysterious compound that was working to do the complete opposite; something that helped protect cells from cancerous changes, reduced the risk of atherosclerosis (the build-up of plaque in the arteries) and, even better, worked to reduce the storage of fat in the body.

This was back in 1978 and it took Professor Mike Pariza and his team at the University of Wisconsin in Madison another six years to fully identify, isolate and name this compound as conjugated linoleic acid (CLA), a substance that occurs naturally in meat and dairy products and which increases when these foods are cooked. (In raw beef, for example, the concentration is 3.1mg per gram of fat, and in a well-done steak, this figure rises to 8.2mg per gram of fat.)

CLA is, in fact, the collective term for the different chemical variations of linoleic acid – one of the omega-6 essential fatty acids, which the body cannot manufacture but must glean from the diet. Ironically, one of the reasons some families may not get enough CLA in the diet is that it is found in some of the foods they have tried for health reasons to cut back on. (Fortunately, CLA can also be sourced from GM-free sunflower and safflower oils.)

To get the full weight-maintenance benefits, you would need to eat the equivalent of 3 grams a day of CLA from either dairy products, vegetable oils or cooked red meat. To meet this intake, the family would need to eat steak for breakfast, lunch and supper. In reality, most people take in just 1 gram, which is why the new CLA supplements – which are safe to give to kids from the age of six* – are walking off the shelves in health stores.

Professor Pariza, a microbiologist, cancer researcher and director of the University's Food Research Institute, who has now

---

*CLA is safe for children but you must give an age-appropriate dose (see page 65 for guidance). Use it to keep your child motivated while you slowly introduce healthier eating habits to help keep the weight off. To learn more about this nutrient, for an up-to-date listing of all current CLA literature, or to contact Professor Mike Pariza in person, visit www.wisc.edu/fri/clarefs.htm.

spent most of his career trying to work out how CLA confers its anti-cancer action, admits he was as sceptical as the next scientist when a picture of the full potential and possible health benefits of CLA started to emerge, not least because there have been no recorded side effects. Having first identified CLA as a potent anti-cancer agent in animal studies, Pariza admits he and his team stumbled across its extraordinary weight-controlling potential when they started to notice that those groups of laboratory mice being fed CLA ate less food and carried significantly less body fat (just 4 per cent compared to a normal average of 14 per cent) than those mice who had the same diets but were not given CLA.

The Pariza team incorporated these findings into their research programme and began to investigate what was going on. They found CLA works in the body in two ways to both **reduce fat** and **increase muscle tone**.

First, it regulates several of the enzymes involved in fat metabolism, including one called lipoprotein lipase which works to break down fat globules in the blood. It increases the activity of this enzyme. At the same time, it reduces the action of a second enzyme, called heparin-releasable lipoprotein lipase, which works to increase the uptake of fats into the fat cells. In other words, it **speeds up fat breakdown** and **blocks fat uptake**.

Secondly, it acts on the way the body uses its fat stores for the production of energy. This process relies on a key vitamin-like nutrient called carnitine and, again, CLA works on a related enzyme, carnitine-palmityl transferase, which controls how quickly muscles can burn off fat.

In clinical trials, CLA has now been shown to bring about an average 20 per cent reduction in body fat if taken for at least three months, and in studies concentrating on body builders, researchers at Kent State University in Ohio showed that taking regular supplements of CLA increased arm girth, boosted lean muscle mass and enhanced overall muscle strength. In other words, it doesn't just keep the fat off, it helps you change your body shape for the better!

What to Do When They Won't Eat

When we hear the words anorexia or bulimia, we imagine the emaciated body of a half-starved teen girl who has become too frightened to eat. Imagine the same thing but turn the clock back and in your mind's eye see a five-year-old girl. Because children as young as five (and even three) are just as likely to be concerned about their weight and their body image as a teenager. Researchers at the Women's Hospital in Boston were understandably horrified when they interviewed 200 five-year-old girls and discovered more than half of them to be preoccupied by their weight and susceptible to body-image distortions. And what all these little girls believed was that the real reason most women want to be thinner was 'so they could get more dates'.

The children had a good understanding of what foods are

considered 'bad' and 'fattening' but thought that dieting meant simply eating more fruits and vegetables; a definition that little girls on this side of the Atlantic echo. When researchers at Liverpool University's Department of Primary Care, for example, wanted to know what schoolgirls aged between twelve and thirteen in this country understood by the term 'healthy eating', they sent out over 140 questionnaires and learned that, again, the most popular definition was 'eating more fruits, vegetables and salads'. For the schoolgirls this also amounted to dieting. The problem with this, of course, is that only those girls trying to lose weight thought they needed to eat these 'healthier' foods.

For some parents, the line dividing dieting and anorexia nervosa – which was only given a medical definition in 1988, long after one of my school pals had died from it – is very fine. If you suspect your daughter or son may be suffering from any of the major eating disorders, don't try to tackle it on your own but get professional help.

At first we were told that anorexia and bulimia were psychological problems, but researchers have now found that sufferers often have chemical imbalances that mirror those of people suffering from clinical depression. In some cases, anorexia has also been linked with a severe zinc deficiency (for more about zinc and supplementation, see page 86).

Here are some tell-tale warning signs that an eating disorder may be developing:

- Noticeable and abnormal weight loss
- An intense fear of gaining weight
- Constant dieting
- Preoccupation with food
- Refusal to eat anything except the tiniest of portions
- Obsession with exercising and working out
- Extra-sensitivity to the cold

If you can't get through to your child on medical grounds, appeal to his or her vanity. This is what conditions like anorexia and bulimia do to the body:

- Erosion of the enamel on the back teeth (from repeated vomiting)
- Hair loss
- Excessive growth of facial or body hair which is a result of not enough protein in the diet
- Periods stopping
- Broken blood vessels in the face
- Swelling of the neck
- Ulcers
- Low blood pressure
- Dizziness
- Weakness
- Death . . . starving the body will cause a deficiency in sodium and potassium, the minerals that play a key role in keeping the heart and heartbeat healthy. Prolonged starvation can cause an irregular heartbeat and cardiac arrest.

The **Eating Disorders Association** runs a nationwide helpline on 01603 621414 which is manned from 9 a.m. to 6.30 p.m., Mondays to Fridays. You can also visit the website at www.edauk.com.

Get Professional Help

I do not recommend a DIY recovery programme for a condition as serious as this. Find a nutritionist or naturopath who can help your child build his or her nutritional profile back to optimum levels. Try the **British Association of Nutritional Therapists** on 0870 6061284. You will be charged £2 for a referral list. The **British Naturopathic Association** on 01458 840072 holds a list of qualified naturopaths who combine nutrition, herbalism and homeopathy in their treatment programmes.

Getting Kids Off the Couch

In America – where one in five adults is 30 per cent overweight and where the number of obese children has doubled in the last twenty years – health experts are now so worried abut this trend that children are being offered free swimming and cycling sessions. That's great, but how are you going to convince the kids to get off their butts and do something more active than reach for the remote control if the parents do nothing more strenuous than raiding the fridge?

My point is that you are going to have to practise what you preach to your kids and that doesn't mean disappearing to the gym three times a week, leaving the video player to babysit them. It doesn't mean taking them with you either. Gym-tots may be a popular crêche substitute among celebrity mums but gym workouts can do more harm than good for kids under fourteen. While the developing body is well equipped to cope with the normal demands of playtime and a moderate amount of aerobic activity, health experts have warned it is not designed for pounding treadmills or lifting heavy weights.

Parents whose kids are involved in a lot of sport, especially football training, may already be familiar with a condition called **Osgood-Schlatter disease** (see page 358) where the growth plates at the top of the shin bone become inflamed following exercise. Another increasingly common problem is *Chondromalacia patellae*, which is the result of an imbalance of muscular strength between the two sides of the knee cap.

A better form of exercise for younger bodies is **yoga** (see page 148), which is designed to build strength and flexibility and improve breathing and body awareness. If your kid thinks yoga is for cissies, show him or her a photo of the popstars Sting or Madonna – both huge Astanga yoga devotees – and ask how cissy they both look. Tell them too that yoga is fast becoming one of the more popular activities among young offenders in prisons!

- **To find kids' yoga classes in your area, write to Lidia Flisek, Body Awareness, c/o 29b Bardolph Road, London N7 0NJ**

Difficult Behaviours and Learning Problems

Ask most parents to list the top three most challenging behavioural disorders a parent may have to face and they will say autism, Attention Deficit Disorder (ADD) and Attention Deficit Hyperactivity Disorder (ADHD). Dyspraxia, which is characterized by a pronounced clumsiness, and dyslexia (see A–Z, page 325), where problems in reading and recognizing letters can make school learning a nightmare, can also affect your child's behaviour in and out of the classroom. What few parents will yet know is that according to neuroscientists investigating what's going wrong in the brains of these kids, there may be no need to give all these disorders different names or even different treatments because, if you bring it all down to the molecular level, what's happening is the exact same biochemical malfunction.

The link between these conditions first came to light when researchers realized very few kids presented with just one or the other disorder and that the overlap between them was high. Between ADHD and dyslexia, for instance, the overlap ranges from 30 to 50 per cent; between ADHD and dyspraxia and between dyslexia and dyspraxia it is 50 per cent. More boys are affected than girls (4:1 with dyspraxia) and if you take all three disorders, ADHD, dyslexia and dyspraxia, one in twenty UK kids currently suffers severe symptoms. Add in those with mild to moderate difficulties and that figure rises to one in ten children. At the moment, if a diagnosis of dyslexia is made, your child would be referred to an educational psychologist; if you were told your child had ADHD you could find yourself at the door of a paediatric psychiatrist, and if the doctor pinpointed dyspraxia, you would be making an appointment with the physiotherapist. And all along it may turn out the person you should be seeing is the family nutritionist.

Instead, and before too long, you'll be dropping your child off at school with Ritalin – the number-one drug (after antibiotics) we now give to our kids. Did you know this drug has been banned in Sweden or that its toxicology is very similar, almost identical, to that of cocaine?

Since the start of the 1900s usage has increased 600-fold, causing a growing number of toxicologists and scientists to ask why we are exploding such a powerful stimulant down the throats of – what? Naughty kids? Especially when, according to cutting-edge research, for some of these kids the solution really could be as simple as changing the diet.

New research is suggesting that all these behavioural and learning problems may be linked to an underlying inability to convert essential fatty acids (EFAs) in the diet into the highly unsaturated fatty acids (HUFAs) which are crucial to healthy brain functioning and, thus, to behaviour and performance. The reason these unsaturated fatty acids are so crucial is simple. The membranes of the brain cells are made up of phospholipids composed of fatty acids. The more unsaturated those fatty acids, the more fluid the membrane and, thus, the more effective the cell-to-cell signalling (see page 238).

There are two key reasons your child's brain may be having a problem. The first is that since the body cannot make essential fatty acids but must rely on dietary intake, your child may simply not be getting enough EFAs in the diet in the first place. The second is that even if he or she does get enough, something may be going wrong with the EFA to HUFA conversion mechanism itself.

Here are just some of the factors which can impair the conversion of EFAs to HUFAs in the body:

- **Saturated, hydrogenated and transfats in the diet all impede the conversion process. What are junk diets rich in? All three.**

- There may be underlying deficiencies in zinc and vitamin B6, both of which play key roles in the conversion process too.
- Any excess of alcohol or coffee will impair this process.
- Smoking will also impair the process.
- Too many stress hormones circulating will have an adverse effect.
- Viral infections may be responsible since viruses can disable the conversion mechanism.
- A history of allergies, including eczema or psoriasis, suggests a link between the conversion process and immune functioning too.
- Being male. The female hormone, oestrogen, helps the body convert EFAs to HUFAs. Conversely, testosterone impedes the enzyme that builds HUFAs.

Signs of essential fatty acid deficiency, which include frequent urination, excessive thirst, dry skin and hair, soft and brittle nails, poor concentration and disturbed sleep patterns, are all symptoms frequently reported by parents of children diagnosed with these now seemingly related disorders.

What to do

Your first step should be to **eliminate salicylate-rich foods** such as **apples, oranges and tomatoes,** which can all exacerbate the problem. What happens is that the salicylates 'displace' the essential fatty acids and get converted to salicylic acid, a substance similar to aspirin which can irritate the stomach and other tissues.

Your second, even more crucial, change should be to supplement the diet with a **high dose (1g/2 tablespoons a day of a liquid supplement) of essential fatty acids** from either unpolluted fish or, if you prefer a vegetarian option, flaxseed oil. If your child dislikes the taste, hide the oil in tomato ketchup or salad dressings and remember, since clinical trials show it can take three months before you see any significant improvements, you will need to be patient.

A number of these children have also been found to have low levels of the brain chemical **serotonin** (see Depression, page 49) so taking the same steps as recommended for depression through both diet and natural medicine to boost production of this feel-good neurotransmitter will help too. Many, especially those aged five to nine, are also low in **zinc** so, again, parents should consider a high-dose daily supplement – **10mg** – of this nutrient as well. Vitamin B12, which works to improve concentration, memory and balance, can also help.

What you should really do, of course, is **talk to a nutritionist** with a special interest in these problems, most of which have also been linked back to the use of antibiotics in the first six months of infancy although nobody can yet explain why. Synthetic food colourings and flavourings (see Food Additives, page 34) have also been linked so try to cut down on your child's intake of these substances too.

- Health professionals and parents looking for more details should contact NS3UK, a nutrition organization with a special interest in child health, which also trains practitioners. Call 01344 360033 or visit the website at www.ns3.co.uk.
- You can also contact the UK's leading research expert in this field in person. Dr Alex Richardson is on alex.richardson@physiol.ox.ac.uk. She believes the body cannot do as good a conversion job of EFAs to HUFAs from flaxseed oils as from fish oils, and when asked recently if her findings have been accepted now by mainstream medicine, she said: 'You just have to wait for these fossils to move on.'
- For more general information and guidance, check out the Dyslexia Research Trust on www.dyslexic.org.uk.

Five-star Tip

Lots of parents report dramatic improvements when they use **Cognis** – one of the combination Australian bush flower remedies. It includes Bush Fuchsia which integrates left- and right-brain function, Paw Paw which will help a child who is feeling overwhelmed by pressures, Sundew which addresses any lack of focus and feelings of being spaced out, and Isopogen which promotes memory (and has been used in Australia for Alzheimer's patients). For more details, contact Ancient Roots on 020 8421 9877, or visit the website at www.ancient-roots.com. Combine this with Nutrition Now's Rhino Actalin Brain Support which also works to restore healthy nerve function and calm the brain. For details, call Victoria Health on 0800 413596.

Homeopathy and Autism

In America – and thanks mostly to the efforts of one determined mother who refused to accept nothing could be done for her autistic son – doctors investigating a link between a hormonal digestive disorder and autism have reported some success with a procedure called the Secretin Challenge Test. Secretin is a hormone which stimulates the pancreas to produce more bicarbonate, which is then used to neutralize the acid contents of the stomach before they are emptied into the alkaline environment of the small intestine.

Injecting secretin into autistic children has been found to improve their language and concentration skills, help them sleep and relate to people better, and counter the facial tics which are another common symptom of autism. The trouble is, there may be long-term side effects. Most doctors refuse to carry out this treatment, and those that do often charge as much as £1,500 a shot.

A better solution, which aims to achieve the same restoration of the role of secretin in the disorder, is a homeopathic one. At the moment several hundred British families who have been testing the remedy for a year or so are reporting mixed but mostly favourable results.

What has surprised researchers is that a homeopathic hormonal remedy can normalize the action of an aberrant hormone. Even better, and even if it only works for a handful of the million autistic children in this country, it costs just £9 for a remedy that will last two months.

Most parents using homeopathic secretin favour the liquid form, which can be added to normal drinks. The recommended daily dose is three drops of the remedy in a little water twice a day. The doses should not be given immediately before or after brushing the child's teeth because the mint in toothpaste can prevent the remedy from working. Parents reporting improvements say they start to see positive changes about two weeks after starting treatment. Changes can continue for another four or five weeks, after which time families report a kind of 'plateau' effect. At this stage, you can reduce or even stop the remedy. However, if the benefits disappear, you will need to restart the daily doses.

Tony Pinkus, managing director of Ainsworths, the homeopathic pharmacy which pioneered the development of this new secretin remedy in the UK, says: 'One advantage of the homeopathic solution to the secretin problem is that the remedy does not introduce any synthetic substance into the body.'

Keith Lovett, a founder member of the Society for the Autistically Handicapped, says the pressure for a homeopathic secretin remedy came from the parents of autistic children themselves: 'There are remedies available, especially in America and Japan, but they tend to mix the secretin with other ingredients, such as herbs, which is not how classical homeopathy works. Parents were asking us about a homeopathic remedy but we were finding homeopaths themselves did not know about secretin or very much about autism. This new remedy has been developed by people who know about both.'

• **Ainsworths can be contacted on 020 7935 5330. For more information about secretin and autism visit the website at www.ainsworths.com. Also visit www.autismuk.co.**

Meningitis: Every Parent's Nightmare

Meningitis is an infection and inflammation of the three meninges – thin membranes that cover the brain and spinal cord. It can be caused by both bacteria and viruses (bacterial meningitis is more life-threatening than viral meningitis) but can be treated by antibiotics if you catch it in time. Viral meningitis tends to occur in local outbreaks, over winter months and in cycles. (This is why sometimes the newspapers seem to be full of headlines screaming about an outbreak while at other times you hear nothing about this disease.)

From the age of eight weeks, the majority of infants and children in the UK are still routinely vaccinated against the HIB micro-organism (see the Vaccine Debate, page 7) which means the most common form of bacterial meningitis is now meningococcal meningitis. (For an explanation about C-strain meningitis, see page 29.)

This is a frightening illness. Babies, children and even adult sufferers can fall sick and worsen rapidly. Their recovery depends on getting the right treatment quickly enough, which can translate as you, the parent, recognizing the symptoms in your child and raising the alarm. What's frightening is that in the early stages you cannot be sure what is causing these symptoms. If that's the case, always assume the worst. It's better being told you over-reacted than experiencing the worst kind of 'if only' after the event.

The symptoms to look out for

- **Drowsiness/stupor**
- **Fever**
- **Oversensitivity to light**

- Vomiting
- Increased crying
- Shivering
- Headache (usually severe)
- Stiff neck and back
- Cold hands and feet
- Rapid breathing
- Stomach pains
- Aching joints
- In the case of C-strain meningitis, a rash (see below)

In very young infants look out for

- A high-pitched cry
- Seizure/convulsions
- Loss of consciousness
- A bulging or 'tight' fontanelle (soft spot)
- A stiff body with jerky movements
- Loss of appetite
- A pale, blotchy skin

The Glass Rash Test

If you see a rash of flat pink or purple blotchy spots appear, and if these don't fade when you press a drinking glass against them, you are dealing with **meningitis C**, where the infection is poisoning the bloodstream. The toxins in the bacteria damage the blood vessels and blood leaks out, causing the blotchy rash. This damage to the blood vessels can then affect the blood supply to major organs, including the liver and kidneys. If these fail, the patient will die.

This strain is more prevalent in teens and older kids living in close proximity such as university halls of residence. If you think there is any possibility you are dealing with this, call the doctor at once. Without prompt medical attention, this disease can be fatal.

When In Doubt . . . Call the Doctor!

If your child shows any of the above symptoms, especially when recovering from a respiratory illness or sore throat, call the doctor. This is a serious infection which, if not treated promptly, could leave your child with a legacy of hearing or visual problems, learning difficulties and even cerebral palsy. But if the right treatment is given early enough, the risk of lasting complications is thankfully low.

Using Natural Medicine to Support Your Child's Recovery

The homeopathic remedies for meningitis are belladonna and aconite. That said, if I was dealing with these symptoms, I would be calling the doctor first and the homeopath second. This is a classic case for a truly complementary and integrated approach, where conventional medicine does what it does best – that is, tackles and treats the acute symptoms of a disease – and then, once your child is out of hospital and home again and the infection has been cleared, natural medicine can do what it does best too, which is to support the body through recovery and restore optimum health in those systems that have been whacked by the infection and the conventional treatments.

The starting place with this kind of support, especially after an infection as debilitating as meningitis, is the immune system. To really boost it, you need to use what many natural health experts describe as the most powerful of all the immune-boosting agents: a Chinese herb called **astragalus** in the West and **huang chi** in Chinese medicine. Rich in minerals and micronutrients, supplements are made from the root of this plant, which is increasingly used by natural healers to stimulate the immune systems of cancer patients after treatment.

Astragalus has been shown, in lab tests, to stimulate the macrophage cells which engulf and destroy foreign invaders, to promote antibody formation by the immune system's B cells and to increase the proliferation of disease-fighting T cells. (For more details on how all these cells work, see the Immune System, page 268.) Do not give astragalus to a child with a fever or high temperature.

Astragalus will also work to strengthen the movements and muscle tone of the digestive tract, which is the second body system you need to support, especially after your child has been given intravenous (IV) antibiotics.

Its third action in the body is to protect the liver, which acts, if you like, as the body's chemical processing plant, and which will also be clearing out toxins following the infection and IV drug treatments. (If meningitis is suspected, doctors will not wait for lab tests to confirm the diagnosis but will administer a heavy-duty antibiotic treatment regimen, which is usually given intravenously for seven days.)

You can buy astragalus from good health stores either in the form of a standardized extract, available as large tablets which you will need to grind into a powder to give to your child, or in tincture form. The best of the tablet brands is **Solgar**. The best of the tinctures is made by **HerbCraft**. If you have trouble sourcing either, call Solgar for local stockists on 01442 890355, or mail-order HerbCraft from Victoria Health on 0800 413596. To support recovery after a meningitis infection, give your child one age-appropriate dose (see Phytomedicine, page 101) three times a day, during the recovery phase* only and for no longer than two weeks.

The B vitamins, which work best when taken together, help the body combat stress and help restore lost energy. Buy a good quality **B complex supplement** and, again, give an age-related dose (for guidance, see Supplements, page 65). Give as directed on the bottle for two weeks once doctors confirm the infection has been cleared.

Once your child is back home recovering, serve nourishing, wholesome foods (avoid highly processed and high-sugar meals) and provide longer-term support to the digestive system by giving him or her a good quality **probiotic** (see Probiotics, page 95) **with Fructooligosaccharides (FOS)**, the natural plant substances which favour and feed those beneficial bacteria that live in the gut where they boost the absorption of nutrients and aid digestion. One of the best combination probiotic products now available here is **Nutrition Now's Rhino FOS and Acidophilus** which you can buy in powder or chewable tablet form. For details, call Victoria Health again (0800 413596).

Quick-fix Treat

Trying to be All Things to All People? Busy mums need the Australian bush flower remedy Black-eyed Susan (I never leave home without my dropper) or, even better, the combination remedy Calm and Clear. To order call Ancient Roots on 020 8421 9877, fax on 020 8950 7733 or visit the excellent website at www.ancient-roots.com.

*Do not use this herb while infection is still present.

Why We Get Bacterial Meningitis

Meningitis may be potentially lethal but the bacterium causing it is weak and cannot survive outside the body for more than a few minutes. In fact, most people are carriers – the bacteria live harmlessly in the mucus at the back of the nose and throat – and have no symptoms at all. But one person in a thousand is susceptible, thanks to a weakened immune system. And when this is the case, the bacteria can pass into the bloodstream, causing meningitis septicaemia (or C-strain meningitis) which is always accompanied by a rash, or into the brain, causing HIB. C-strain meningitis is also a bacterial strain and while HIB causes most harm in babies and kids under four, C-strain is most harmful to older children and is responsible for recent teen deaths from meningitis in the UK.

The genetically modified C-strain vaccine is still very new – it was only introduced in the UK in the autumn of 1999. Since then, some health experts have expressed concern about possible side effects, including juvenile arthritis.

Quick-fix Treat

Lose 10 Years in a Week! I usually hate the word 'miracle' – especially on skin creams – but I make an exception for Seven Wonders Miracle Lotion, an American-formulated skin cream which works magic on all skin types. Rich in seven natural and essential oils plus fourteen fabulous herbs, including goldenseal and sage, this is the one my 'mean gene' (the one that wants me to keep the really good stuff to myself) doesn't want to tell you about. It costs just £9.95. Mail-order from Ancient Roots on 020 8421 9877. Use on your face and watch the wrinkles fade overnight. Try it – I promise, you'll love me for ever!

Food Additives

Remember E numbers? When parents got wise to the potential health hazards of many of the additives being added to foods and labelled with E numbers, food makers simply switched back to the long chemical names. True, lots of these chemicals sound pretty unsavoury, but how many busy mums and dads really have time to stop in the supermarket and start reading food labels? Very few – which is just what the manufacturers rely on.

According to government estimates, your child will have consumed the equivalent of almost half a pound (about 250g) of artificial colourings by the age of thirteen. That's almost 50mg – milligrams – of chemical dye every day. And if your child eats a lot of processed food, that figure can be as high as 146mg a day. These figures exclude caramels – colourings made with ammonia – that are present in colas, chocolate, confectionery, snack foods, biscuits, cereals and cakes. Add in these additives and your children could be eating the equivalent of three-quarters of a pound (about 375g) of artificial colourings a year.

Children are more vulnerable to the harmful effects of additives than any other sector of the population yet the fact is that almost all your children's favourite foods – the ones you like too, for their convenience – are bursting with additives. Additive, by the way, means any chemical that is added to food or any other everyday item, such as shampoo and detergent, by the manufacturer. (Any chemical used before this stage, such as pesticides or herbicides, is not included.)

As an experiment, I recently allowed my five-year-old daughter to choose five items that caught her eye in the supermarket. The following items are what she chose:

- Fish fingers (of course!)
- Cheese-flavoured crisps
- A sugar-free jelly (blackcurrant flavour)
- Those terrible cheese strings (show me a kid that doesn't love these)
- A chow-mein-flavoured pot noodle (don't ask!)

All bright, fun-looking foods that any kids aged five to fifteen would similarly make a beeline for. And all laden with potentially sickening additives. And had I not binned most of them here's what my daughter would really have been eating:

- **Fish fingers** contain modified maize starch which is a thickening and binding agent: high in calories and low in nutritional value. In other words, empty bulk. The starch is treated with various chemicals to modify it. Two of these chemicals, epichlorohydrin and propylene oxide, are suspected of causing genetic mutations and cancer. The thing is, you won't know if they've been used because the label doesn't have to tell you. These fish fingers also contained 'natural colours curcumin and paprika'. Curcumin, which is also known as E100, is found in lots of foods kids love, including biscuits and sweets. It can damage animal genes.

- **Cheese-flavoured crisps** contain a flavouring agent called E621. You will know this better as monosodium glutamate (MSG). This crosses the blood–brain barrier and acts as a neuro-toxin. (It has now been withdrawn from baby-food products in America, after animal tests showed doses equivalent to those being used in these foods had the potential to cause brain damage.) This is the same ingredient that is heavily used in western Chinese take-away restaurants. In large amounts, it has been shown to cause a state of intoxication. Milder symptoms can include a flushed face and foggy mind. It can also trigger migraine headaches – a common reaction now known as Chinese Restaurant Syndrome.

These harmless-looking crisps, which are so clearly targeted at kids, also contain E160(b), or the yellow food colouring annatto, which can cause an allergic reaction in susceptible individuals. Another tasty E number is E635 – a mixture of E627 and E631 – which is used to cut down on more expensive ingredients and which is banned in baby and infant foods.

- **Sugar-free jelly** – are you impressed she chose a healthy sugar-free variety? Don't be. It's the first of her five foods that went into the rubbish bin. The reason there's no real sugar in it is that the jelly is packed with artificial sweeteners aspartame and acesulfame K, neither of which have E numbers (see the section on Keeping Them Sweet, pages 44–8).

  Since she chose blackcurrant 'flavour' her jelly also contains Green S, a green colouring that was banned in the UK before it got the green light from the EU. Made from coal-tar dye (also known as an azo dye), it can cause allergic reactions, but it can also be found in 'health' drinks. Carmosine is a red colouring also present and made from coal-tar but even worse than azo dye. A suspected carcinogen, it can also reduce fertility in women. (To make a jelly that really is naturally sweet and healthy, see Raspberry Jelly Secrets, page 218).

- **Cheese strings** – don't be misled into thinking the words 'cheese flavour' have much to do with cheese. Over nine out of ten food additives are 'flavours'. Flavours are not subject to any regulations or control and the only person who'll be able to tell you what any flavour actually is will be the food technologist who dreamt it up. Nobody will even admit how many flavours are now used in British food. Some say 3,000. Others say twice that number. The fact is, there is no toxicity data on most of these flavouring agents. So, if you take nothing else from this book, at least know that when a food says cheese or strawberry or beef 'flavour', the chance of it having had a real encounter with a real food is non-existent.

The one additive we can identify in this food is E160(b) or annatto; the yellow food colouring that was also present in her crisps.

- **Pot noodles – chow-mein flavour** – back to that word 'flavour', which means it's anyone's guess what she might have been eating here. This is yet another of those 'trade secrets' the food manufacturers are allowed to keep. So let's see what we can identify. Well, there's E621, which we've already seen from her crisps is the flavour enhancer monosodium glutamate (MSG), and there's E635, which again cropped up in the crisps and which is, in fact, sodium 5-ribonucleotide. (Maybe we should be relieved they didn't use E631, sodium 5-inosinate, which is prepared from animal muscle waste and used in, among other things, instant soups.) There's curcumin or E100 again (remember that from the fish fingers?) and there's another ingredient called maltodextrin which is a version of the sugar maltose but so highly refined there's nothing natural left. This, along with sucrose, dextrose, fructose and lactose, is one of the chemicals any family eating the typical western diet is going to be eating a lot of, and as with those other sugars high consumption is responsible for obesity in kids and type II (adult-onset) diabetes and heart disease in their parents.

Banned Additives

The Food Advisory Committee (which used to be the Food Additives and Contaminants Committee) has now spent several years considering the merits or otherwise of additives in foods for babies and young children. It has yet to publish any official report but, in the meantime, the government and European officials have banned some substances.

Here are some additives that have been banned from foods that are specially prepared for babies and young children:

- E310 (propyl gallate)
- E311 (octyl gallate)
- E312 (dodecyl gallate)
- E320 (butylated hydroxyanisole)
- E321 (butylated hydroxytoluene)

Here are some of the foods you'll find them in:

- Squash drinks
- Instant puddings
- Instant mash

- Some cereals
- Sweets
- Crisps
- Biscuits
- Mousses
- Cakes

All foods mums and dads are just as likely to serve to kids because, as every parent knows, children don't just eat foods that have been 'specially prepared for kids'. They eat lots of different foods and they eats lots of those 'adult' foods, such as crisps and soft drinks, that contain additives that have been banned for kids.

At-a-Glance Guide to 20 of the Worst Additives You Should Avoid

Additives which have been approved by the EEC have an E number. Those not approved by the EEC but allowed by the UK have a number but no E. Remember, too, the words 'free from artificial flavourings, colourings and preservatives' might not be as reassuring as they are intended to be. Did you know that some flavourings can be synthesized but called 'natural' (and therefore not counted as an additive) if their chemical structure is the same as the natural flavour? If you are wondering why this is a problem, sharing a chemical structure with a natural product is no guarantee that the artificial substance will act in the body in the same way as the natural one.

For instance, when you read 'caramel flavouring' you will think of the deliberately burnt sugar often used in good old-fashioned baking. What you won't think of is ammonia or sulphite, which is what these agents are actually derived from. If you start reading food labels and begin to think you're walking into a jungle of deliberately misleading jargon, you'll be right! Additives cover colourings, preservatives, antioxidants, sweeteners, emulsifiers, stabilizers, thickeners and binding agents.

E100 Curcumin: Found in fish fingers, yoghurts and sweets and linked to gene damage in animal tests.

E107 Yellow 2G: A yellow colouring found in chocolate, sweets and sauces which is a suspected carcinogen (cancer-causing agent). Also adversely affected the kidneys in animal trials.

E110 Sunset Yellow: Found in hundreds of foods, including yoghurts, jams, cakes and ice cream. Suspected carcinogen that can make some people allergic to sunlight.

E122 Azo Dye: Red colouring found in jams, ice cream, soups and jellies. Also present in 'blackcurrant'-flavoured 'health' drinks. Another suspected carcinogen.

E128 Red 2G: Another azo dye and red colouring used to coat fish fingers, sausages, Scotch eggs and chocolate-flavour instant whips. Breaks down to Red 10B which is thought to cause chromosomal damage.

E131 Patent Blue V: What's a blue colouring doing in peas? Beats me but check anyway. A suspected carcinogen which can cause nausea and shaking in sensitive individuals.

E133 Brilliant Blue: Found in sparkling fruit drinks and apple and blackcurrant drinks. Can cause an allergic reaction.

E150 Caramels: Almost all are made from ammonia and found in hundreds of foods from hamburgers to chocolate ice cream and colas. Some of the many different forms are mutagenic (causing damage or mutations to the genetic material) but described as 'natural' on labels.

E153 Carbon Black: Linked with skin cancer in workers handling large amounts but still present in chocolate-flavoured coatings, choc ices and chocolate-flavoured dessert mixes.

E154 Kipper Brown: Found in foods as varied as sausages and sweets. Now branded carcinogenic and banned in several countries.

E249–E252 The Nitrite Chemicals: Curing agents used in sausages, hot dogs, salami, bacon, pâté, frozen pizzas and Edam cheese. Described as 'some of the most worrying additives' currently used. Banned in food for babies, they can be converted to nitrates which then combine with other food or drugs in the stomach to form cancer-causing agents. They can also prevent the uptake of oxygen by the blood.

E407 Carrageenan Irish Moss (seaweed extract): Used in cakes, biscuits, ice creams, jellies and cheese spreads; permitted in baby foods. Labelled as 'natural' but carcinogenic in animals.

E422 Glycerol: A sweetener used in chewing gum and other sweets. Adverse effects can include nausea, headache and thirst. May also cause bowel disturbances.

432–436 The Polyoxyethylene Sorbitan Chemicals: Used as wetting agents in agricultural sprays, these chemicals increase the absorption of other pollutants in the body. Suspected carcinogens, too, they were banned by the EEC in 1984.

E450(b) The Tri- and Polyphosphate Chemicals: Added to meat to make it take up water to increase the weight (and thus the price) at no extra cost to the manufacturer. Can interfere with digestive enzymes.

E466 Carboxymethyl Cellulose Sodium Salt: A bulking agent found in hot dogs, burgers, ice creams, dessert toppings, orange and lemon drinks and lunchbox juices in a carton. A suspected carcinogen which can cause stomach bloating and gas.

Isomalt: An unnumbered additive. It is a mix of sugars that has been banned in baby and infant foods but may be present in the 'adult' foods children are also eating.

Extract of Quillaia: A frothing agent used in soft drinks, this additive has been linked to intestinal damage.

Aspartame: 200 times sweeter than sugar and not permitted in foods for babies and young children. Breaks down into substances which enhance the stimulatory effect of flavourings such as MSG, adversely affecting the nervous system. A suspected carcinogen. (See pages 44–5.)

Xylitol: Approved by the World Health Organization (WHO) as a sugar substitute against tooth decay – and found in some chewing gums – this additive, which is more often used in food as a bulk sweetener, is toxic to the brain, liver and urinary passages when injected in high doses. It can also cause diarrhoea when eaten.

Remember, all these additives are found in many more than the foods listed here.

*****
Five-star Tip

Invest in a copy of *Additives – Your Complete Survival Guide* (published by Century and edited by Felicity Lawrence), which is brilliant. It has a useful alphabetical list of additives (pages 229–36) and not only teaches you how to read and 'interpret' food labels but devotes a whole chapter to how and why the health of our kids is at very real risk from the foods they eat.

Testing for Toxicity

Everything is a poison . . . in the wrong doses. What this means is that no chemical is toxic when the dose is low enough and all chemicals are poisonous when the dose is too high. It also means too much salt, too much sugar and even too many organic carrots can be bad for your child's health. The question, then, is who decides how much is too much?

Food additives and preservatives undergo exhaustive testing individually, with laboratory animals being given huge doses of a single additive to test for toxicity. What nobody can ever test for is what really happens when all the different additives in a food break down and interact with each other in your body. You will never find a commercial food product that contains just one chemical yet very few studies acknowledge this risk. One that did was reported in the *Journal of Food Science*. The researchers showed that when laboratory rats were given a single additive in their food, there were no notable adverse effects. When two additives were combined, the rats sickened and died. When all three additives were given, all the rats were dead in a fortnight.

*****

Five-star Tip

Check beauty and personal care products for chemical ingredients too. For alternatives, read the labels in health stores and contact the **Green People Company** (01403 822531), which was established by biochemist Charlotte Vontz when she wanted chemical-free products, including shampoos, toothpastes and suncreams, for her own young family.

Keeping Them Sweet

I was deeply shocked when I began to research children's nutritional supplements and discovered that the majority contain artificial sweeteners, including aspartame, which you might know better as Nutrasweet. What on earth is aspartame doing in dietary supplements that are on sale in so-called health stores?

Aspartame, which is two hundred times sweeter than sugar, has now been linked to a range of health problems in kids, from headaches to hyperactivity. The list for adults too includes depression, memory loss, rashes, gastrointestinal problems and, in extreme cases, even seizures and double vision. The Aspartame Information group (funded by artificial sweetener companies) will tell worried parents that every clinical trial that has concluded that aspartame might not be such a good thing to pour down the necks of our kids was in some way deeply flawed.

I say read on.

Aspartame was discovered in 1965 during research to identify new ulcer drugs. It is made up of phenylalanine, aspartic acid and methanol (or wood alcohol), which breaks down in the body into formaldehyde and is known to be poisonous even in small amounts. Aspartic acid, by the way, is the neurotransmitter or brain chemical which some researchers have suggested can cause brain lesions by literally overexciting some brain cells to death. Who are those most at risk? Children and the elderly whose protective blood–brain barrier may not be fully functional.

The only contraindication or warning you will be given about aspartame – which is now present in over a thousand products, from breath mints to yoghurts – is not to give it to anyone who suffers from a rare condition called phenylketonuria (PKU). Sufferers of this condition, which affects about one in 15,000 of the population, lack the enzyme that the body needs to convert phenylalanine into another amino acid, called tyrosine. As a result, high levels of phenylalanine can accumulate and cause brain damage. Yet aspartame is the very chemical that American scientists, writing in the *Journal of Neuropathy and Experimental Neurology* at the end of the 1990s, suggested could be to blame for not only a dramatic and sustained increase in the number of brain tumours being reported in the US, but an increase in the malignancy of those tumours too.

Other Sweet Nothings . . .

Aspartame is not, of course, the only artificial sweetener often hiding in both sweet and savoury foods. Get into the habit of checking food labels (and health-food supplements) for aspartame but watch out for other artificial sweeteners too. The names to avoid, where possible, include: **acesulfame, xylitol, mannitol (E421), sorbitol (E420), sorbitol syrup (E420), glycerol (E422), isomalt, thaumatin** and **saccharin**.

If you are worried about artificial sweeteners (or other additives) and want to know more, or believe your child may be suffering side effects linked to using them, contact the **Additives Survivors' Network** at their website www.additivesout.org.uk or by e-mail to geoff.brewer@clara.net.

The Real Thing: Sugar

Sugar in all its guises, including **dextrose, fructose, lactose** and **maltose**, is officially considered a food, rather than an additive, but sugars are now so highly refined that in truth they are often pure chemicals with none of their original biological nature. They may not carry E numbers but their use in a wide range of foods, both sweet and savoury, has had devastating effects on our health. Eating high levels of all these sugars causes tooth decay and obesity in kids and is linked to adult-onset diabetes and heart disease in later life.

The Alternatives: Natural Sweeteners

Our body needs sugar to fuel it, to feed its tissues and to produce energy. In healthy foods, the sugar is properly balanced with minerals and other health-promoting nutrients. In processed and other junk foods, the sugar has been highly refined and there is no natural balance left. This type of sugar hits the bloodstream fast to give an energy high but there is a price to pay. The sudden influx of sugar in large amounts is a shock to the stomach and the pancreas. The body responds by creating a more acid environment, in which minerals and other nutrients are then more quickly used. When this happens, a hard-to-break cycle of sugar cravings starts up. Too much sugar in the system can also adversely affect the body's absorption of calcium from the diet. When this happens, the tissues simply steal the calcium they need from the bones.

The best sources of natural sugar are complex carbohydrate foods such as grains, vegetables and legumes, all of which start to taste sweeter the longer you chew them. If your kids are craving something sweet, offer a snack of organic fruit or, if there is no underlying allergy, almond nuts or coconut flesh. The sweetest vegetables include button mushrooms, carrots, cabbage, cucumber, courgettes, potatoes, shiitake mushrooms, sweet potato and squash. Cooking, especially roasting, increases their sweetness and the more you can serve these foods and move away from the refined sugars your family has become used to, the sooner you can help them all beat unhealthy sugar cravings.

If you want to sweeten dishes at home, you can use the following foods:

Honey: It may have more calories per teaspoon than white sugar but honey is a whole lot healthier. It contains minerals and enzymes, and doesn't disrupt the body's own mineral balance in the way that sugar does. It's sweeter than sugar too. Unheated honey can also help dry excess mucus in kids with runny noses and chesty coughs. Honey is also a good source of fructooligosaccharides (FOS) – natural sugars which help keep digestion healthy.

Date juice and fruit syrups: Sweeter and more concentrated than the fresh fruits.

Maple syrup: This boiled-down sugar extracted from maple tree sap is the favourite in our household.

Molasses: This thick, sticky syrup has a very strong flavour. The first time I used it on porridge I had to abandon the whole bowl – so use sparingly.

Amasake: Made from fermented rice and on sale in good health stores, this is the healthiest of all the natural sweeteners. It contains less than 40 per cent maltose, which is only a third as sweet as white sugar and not as highly processed.

Rice syrup or barley malt: Both natural sweeteners and both less destructive to the body's natural mineral balance than more refined sugars. Again, they are made from the fermented grains.

The Stevia Story

A year or so ago, there was a delicious, safe and widely available alternative to artificial sweeteners on sale in good health stores – a herb called **Stevia** – but since this has now been banned from over-the-counter sales here (and I am still trying to find out exactly why) you will have to find an 'alternative' alternative.

Stevia was first banned in America in 1991 when the FDA ruled it was an unsafe food additive. Their two, somewhat lame and largely unsubstantiated concerns were that it might have a contraceptive effect and that in susceptible individuals it might trigger low blood-sugar levels. The FDA secured an import ban which was then lifted after much lobbying by the American Herbal Products Association. In the US today, Stevia can now be sold as a dietary supplement again, but not as a sweetener.

So get this . . . in the US, Stevia is deemed safe as a dietary supplement but unsafe as a food additive. If you think the profit margins of the artificial sweetener giants may have had a hand in this bizarre double-standard, you might want to contact the American experts at Mission-Possible-USA@Altavista.net and allow yourself to be further enlightened.

Quick-fix Treat

Beat Morning Tiredness This is usually a sign of a blood-sugar imbalance exacerbated by stimulants like that get-up-and-go morning coffee or well-deserved nightcap! This kind of tiredness also signals a deficiency in those minerals crucial for the production of glucose, which is then converted into energy by the body's cells. These include all the B vitamins, so take a good B complex plus chromium and co-enzyme Q10. Take a good multisupplement to provide 200mcg of chromium, which will help rebalance blood sugars, and the equivalent of 100mg of CoQ10 for more energy.

Depression in Childhood

According to studies of 'mood disorders' in children and adolescents, an alarming 7 to 14 per cent of all kids will experience an episode of major depression before the age of fifteen. If you think this cannot be true and someone, somewhere must be exaggerating, consider this: in America, in just twelve months from 1995 to 1996, the number of prescriptions for the adult antidepressant Prozac being handed out to kids aged six to twelve rose by a staggering 209 per cent. That's right. Kids as young as six are being given antidepressants. Here, the first ever nationwide survey of the mental health of children and adolescents was only recently commissioned jointly by the Department of Health, the Scottish Office and the Welsh Office and carried out by the Social Survey Division of the National Statistics Office. Again, researchers were shocked to discover at least one in ten kids aged five to fifteen were suffering from some kind of mental disorder, especially depression. And again, these kids are being given antidepressant drugs that were only introduced into adult psychiatric practice in the 1980s.

What to do

In America, the best-selling herbal antidepressant, St John's wort, is suffering something of a backlash – critics argue the body would respond better to a mood-boosting agent that more closely resembles chemicals already made in the body and not something that remains alien to it – and so natural-health consumers are looking for other ways to control mood swings and depression.

The nutrient emerging as the favourite – despite its high cost – is called **SAMe (pronounced Sammy)**. Already prescribed as an antidepressant in the fourteen different countries where it has been approved, it has proved so popular in the US since its launch there at the end of the 1990s that it now ranks twenty-fifth among the 13,000-or-so supplements on sale in health stores in that country. SAMe – short for S-adenosylmethionine – is neither a herb nor a hormone. It is a molecule which all living cells produce and it is said to be vital to the health of all tissues and organs, including the brain, where it plays a key role in the regulation of the neurotransmitters. These, in turn, control the production of feel-good brain chemicals such as serotonin and dopamine.

This works through a process called methylation which occurs a billion times a second throughout the body, affecting all systems from the developing tissues of the foetus in its mother's womb to the maintenance of adult cell membranes. Biochemists stress the importance of methylation – where a molecule donates a methyl group to an adjacent molecule – and warn that without it, there would be no life. Lots of molecules can do this but SAMe is said to be the most active of all the methyl donors.

Levels of SAMe decline with age – kids usually have around seven times more than their parents – but what is still not clear is how SAMe works. One theory is that it regulates the biochemistry and breakdown of brain chemicals. Another is that it makes the cell receptor sites these chemicals latch onto in the brain even more responsive. The clinical evidence for SAMe is small (just forty trials involving 1,400 patients to date) but persuasive. Nobody is claiming this molecule is more effective than the conventional drugs for controlling depression, but it has been shown to be less toxic, with a mild stomach upset in a handful of patients documented as the only serious reaction to date.

It is safe to give to kids over twelve but do not exceed a daily dose of 200mg. SAMe is still very expensive (twenty tablets can cost over £50) but if it works and has fewer side effects than conventional antidepressants, then for families who can afford it, it will be well worth discussing with their healthcare practitioners. If you do decide to switch, under proper medical supervision, you can mail-order SAMe from **Revital** on 0800 252875.

The body makes SAMe from methionine, an amino acid provided in protein-rich and other foods including yoghurt, eggs, ham, apples, pineapple, lentils and pork. Methionine works in the body to deactivate histamine, high levels of which have also been linked with depression and schizophrenia in adults. **Vitamin C** has a strong antihistamine action in the body too, so make sure any child who is suffering any kind of mood disorder is getting enough of this important antioxidant (for correct dosage levels, see Supplements, page 73).

Another amino acid which can help lift depression is glutamine, sold in supplement form as **L-glutamine**. It can cross the protective blood–brain barrier and so has become known as a potent brain fuel. Lots of foods contain glutamine – spinach and parsley are both good sources – but this nutrient is easily destroyed by cooking. You must not give this supplement to anyone with a liver disorder or kidney problems, and you must make sure you don't confuse it with other, similar-sounding substances such as glutamic acid, glutamate or gluten, which are not the same and have completely different actions in the body.

You can also use diet to boost serotonin levels. For this, you need to take a step back in the biochemistry of the brain. Serotonin is made from **vitamin B6** (see page 70) and a common amino acid called **tryptophan** which is found in lots of foods, from eggs to broccoli, and sweet potato to watercress. It is present, too, in chicken, fish, milk, cauliflower, nuts, soybeans and cottage cheese, and feeding your family more of all these will help improve mood. If this is too hit-and-miss for you, then **Country Life** makes a herbal mood booster that features the stable supplement form of tryptophan which is called **5-HTP**. It also contains **kava kava** (a herb which should be called 'calmer,

calmer'), **passionflower** and **Siberian ginseng**. The latter works to support stressed adrenal glands and boost energy levels, which are usually low in kids and adults suffering from depression. This is a more affordable supplement too: 60 capsules cost around £15.45. To find a stockist near you, call Country Life on 020 8614 1411. Do not give this supplement to children under twelve. For older kids, give an age-appropriate dose.

A good B-complex supplement will help the body cope with the stress of depression and provide the vitamin B6 it needs to boost the production of serotonin. **Biocare's B Complex** is excellent: 60 veggie capsules cost £9.65. If you need to mail-order, call the company direct on 0121 433 3727. Magnesium will also help to lift a low mood. For an age-appropriate dose, see page 79.

Natural Mood Boosters

Safer by far than adult prescription drugs for children suffering from depression are the essential fatty acids (EFAs), which many experts, from neurochemists to molecular geneticists, now believe may play a key role in regulating brain chemicals and banishing mood disorders. Describing the results of preliminary trials using EFAs to treat depression in children as 'remarkable' (not least because previously untreatable cases appeared to go into complete remission), nutritionists and doctors with an interest in this field are now calling for more research.

What we know is that the membranes of brain cells are made up largely of phospholipids, each containing two types of fatty acids, which help determine the action of other chemicals and nutrients in the brain. So-called 'free' fatty acids, which are not part of the cell structure, are also crucial in cell signalling (see pages 237–42).

Until we have more research, it will be up to parents to choose which route they want to go. But I know if it was my daughter, I would not want her taking antidepressants either now or as an adult, and so I would be using a high dose (1g a day) of essential fatty acids, which bring so many other health benefits too.

- **If you want to supplement your child's diet with essential fatty acids (EFAs), give the equivalent of 1g a day, or 2 table-spoons if using a liquid blend. You can use a mixed blend of oils, cod liver oil or, if you prefer a vegetarian source, flaxseed oil. I like Omega Nutrition's Essential Balance Jnr from Higher Nature (01435 882880).**

Quick-fix Treat

Float Off . . . An hour's float is reckoned to be the equivalent of six hours' deep sleep. Even better, US basketball teams who acquired float tanks reportedly shot up the league tables and never looked back, so making time to float can improve your performance at home and at work. Ask for details at your local health spa, and if they don't have a tank yet, ask why not. To find a nearby tank, check out www.floatworks.com. Until you find one, try the next best thing. Alka Bath contains sea salt, minerals and sodium bicarbonate. It costs £14.95 for 750g, which should last several months, and is only available from Best Care Products. Mail-order on 01342 410303 and add £2 p&p.

Chronic Fatigue Syndrome (CFS)

What's happening here? The honest answer is nobody knows. This is a complex condition likely to be caused by a number of seemingly unrelated triggers, from prolonged emotional stress, which often appears to be a key cause, to a relatively common viral infection that most other kids can shake off or live with. What we do know is that CFS affects substantially more females (85 per cent of sufferers) than males, and is more likely to strike both people who have an ongoing history of allergies and over-achievers who set high standards for themselves. It is not contagious and, unlike conditions which are, is not spread to sexual partners or via intravenous drug use.

Rare in children under twelve, CFS starts to emerge in adolescents, who suffer the same range of debilitating symptoms as adults. These include: **multi-joint pain without swelling or redness, a sore throat, tender lymph nodes, muscle pain, disturbed sleep, headaches, poor concentration** and a **poor short-term memory.** In 1994, and after enormous debate, doctors agreed to make a diagnosis of Chronic Fatigue Syndrome only if the patient was suffering from four or more of the above symptoms and only if these symptoms did not pre-date the onset of the disease. To satisfy this new definition of CFS, the patient also has to have suffered from a chronic fatigue that tests prove is not being caused by any other clinical condition and which has lasted for at least six months.

What is clear – and this is why there is no one thing you can do to make sure your child is protected – is that no matter how many times researchers try to find a single cause for this complaint, they are always left having to conclude that while theories about immune impairment and viral infection persist, the evidence seems to point to a lot of different factors, probably including immune malfunction and, as a result, a lingering viral infection at work.

What to Do

Exercise may be the last thing your CFS child feels like doing but any form of aerobic exercise, from walking to swimming, will help to greatly reduce the symptoms. The best way to motivate anyone to do something is to do it with them so don't send them off swimming, go along too.

Kids who have CFS are highly sensitive to environmental and other pollutants (see Additives, page 34). Help the body clear out the free-radical molecules that are a result of the pollutants they may be breathing in or ingesting in processed foods by giving them one of the highly active bioflavonoid supplements. The antioxidant action of **grapeseed extract**, for example, is fifty times stronger than vitamin E and twenty times stronger than vitamin C. Solgar makes a 100mg extract which costs £19.05 for 30 tablets. Give your CFS teenager one a day and switch, whenever possible, to an organic diet to cut down on pollutants in food.

The first enzyme involved in energy production in the body is nicotininamide adenine dinucleotide – **NADH** – which is also known as **co-enzyme 1**. Enzymes are proteins that trigger chemical changes in the body, and NADH, which is a derivative of nicotine, is so important that it is found in all living cells. The only supplement brand that has undergone clinical trials in the US or here is **FSC's NADH**, which is on sale in the GNC high street health stores. Athletes report that NADH makes them feel stronger and more energized. You need to give this supplement, which can also boost concentration levels, half an hour before eating and to limit your CFS patient to no more than two tablets a day.

The second enzyme that plays a key role in energy production in all cells is **co-enzyme Q10 (CoQ10)**. Biocare make a liquid supplement called **Vitasorb** which is suitable for kids (30ml costs £13.35). Mail-order on 0121 433 3727 and remember, ten drops will provide the equivalent of 10mg.

Siberian ginseng is an adaptogen (see page 111), which supports and helps all systems of the body resist stress, infection and sickness. Since CFS patients have also been found to have lower blood levels of the stress hormone cortisol (this is the hormone pumped out by the adrenal glands, which regulate the body's fight-or-flight response to stress) then stress is likely to be playing a role in this condition too. This herb is now widely on sale in good health stores. Give an age-related dosage.

Finally, build a healthy digestive system by giving a good quality **probiotic** – a supplement made up of replacement live bacteria to reinforce levels of those bacteria that aid digestion – together with a **prebiotic**, usually the nutrient FOS, which these bacteria thrive on. (For a detailed explanation on how these work together, see pages 95–9.)

Quick-fix Treat

Float in Rose Petals When I discovered the delicious Lotus Emporium herbal range, I thought I had died and gone to heaven. The Tao Milk Bath includes soothing chamomile, lavender and geranium and a scattering of teeny dried rosebuds. Add to the bath or add water to make a paste which works as a cleansing facemask. To mail-order, call the company direct on 01225 448011. Buy one for yourself, one for a friend and, while you're on the phone, ask about the range of shamanic incense preparations.

The Viral Connection

What we do now know is that in 40 per cent of cases of CFS there is a proven link with an infection by the Epstein-Barr virus (EBV). Although a minority, 40 per cent remains a significant proportion, not least because researchers know that, depending on the tests being used, a number of individuals – up to 15 per cent – who have had the EBV infection will still test negatively for it. If you add the two percentages together, then there could be a link in the majority of sufferers.

EBV is responsible for the typically teenage infection we know as glandular fever – also known as 'kissing disease' since in healthy people the virus is shed in their oral secretions. A member of the herpes family of viruses, it has the same ability to remain dormant in the body long after the primary infection. It 'hides' in the salivary glands and the B-cells of the immune system, where, unless something goes wrong, it can usually be kept in check by the other immune system cells.

The question for CFS sufferers is what has gone so badly wrong that the virus has been able to reactivate itself, and is this the sole reason for their symptoms or is there something else going on too?

The humble hedgerow **elderberry** has antiviral properties and acts specifically against the herpes viruses, especially the Epstein-Barr relative. The way it works is that the active ingredients inhibit or block the virus's replication mechanism. It has strong antioxidant properties, too, which protect the body from free-radical damage, and it is used as an immune system tonic to return the immune system to optimum functioning, so even if you don't know whether your child has had a viral infection, giving this herb will still help.

- **Solgar makes a supplement that combines a standardized elderberry extract (150mg) with the equivalent dosage of powdered raw herb.**

PART TWO

Natural Medicine

Introduction

Walk into any high-street health store and the chances are, unless you've done your homework and know exactly where to look and what to ask for, you'll walk straight out again. This is the section that has done that homework for you.

Maybe you've decided you want to use echinacea to boost your child's immune system. An excellent choice. The trouble is, how do you know which brand and which version to buy? Should you ask for a tincture, a throat lozenge or a tea? What does it mean when the label says standardized extract? And even when you've figured all that out, how do you know how much of an adult formulation you can safely give to a child?

This is the section that answers all those questions and more. You'll learn about all the major nutrients the body needs and how to spot the tell-tale signs of a deficiency in any of them in your own family. You'll find out all about synergy – how you can use nutrients which enhance each other's action in the body together for more effect – and how some of the most powerful natural agents you can use to protect your children from problems as wide-ranging as asthma and erratic and painful periods are in the strange-looking Asian mushrooms now on sale in supermarkets and in supplements.

You probably already try hard to get your kids to eat well and choose healthy foods, and you may be wondering why on earth children would need additional minerals and vitamins. The reason – and sadly, the reality – is that as parents we can only do so much to influence the eating choices our kids are making. And once they start school, that choice for most of their waking hours is out of our hands. Sure, you send them off to school with a healthy lunchbox, but how much gets eaten and how much ends up in the bin or exchanged for something you'd rather they didn't eat?

Smart nutrition can make your kids smarter too. When researchers at the California State University tested the IQs of schoolchildren between the ages of six and twelve, they found those given a daily multisupplement gained an average of 2.5 points on the IQ scales. Even more impressive, those pupils who were noted to be poorly nourished at the start of the study gained a staggering 15 points, leading the scientists to conclude that parents whose kids are not doing so well at school could do a lot worse than check their children's nutritional status and correct any deficiencies or hidden imbalances.

If you're a closet herbalist you'll learn in this section how easy it is to use compresses, poultices and even herbal teas to promote health and treat specific conditions. If you want to learn more about DIY home healing, there's a section on aromatherapy and essential oils, and lots of tips on how and when to use them, plus clear advice on which ones to avoid with youngsters. In this part of the book, you'll also be introduced to a new range of flower essences so contemporary and powerful you'll wonder why nobody's ever even told you about them before (it's because they are new to the UK) and you'll find out how impressive but little-known hands-on treatments such as the Bowen or Metamorphic Techniques get fabulous and lasting results with kids.

If you've ever watched very small children at play, you'll see how they twist and roll and bend their little bodies to work every muscle group and keep their spines flexible. They are relaxed and open and confident with their bodies. So what do we then do? Send them to school to sit on little hard chairs where their bodies start to develop the first signs of stiffness, which you will read more about in this part of the book.

The good news is that the human body is very forgiving and so it won't take too much effort on your (or their) part to regain that earlier flexibility and strength, as long as you know what you are doing. And what you will be doing is yoga for kids, which you are going to enjoy just as much as they do. As a yoga teacher, I've devised a simple but effective thirty-minute lesson you can do with all the kids at home. It's safe, it's easy and it's fun as well as healthy. Try it and I bet the kids like it so much, they'll be nagging you for more, in which case you'll need to find a teacher locally (and this book is packed with contact details to help you find the right practitioners) or buy the books I have recommended as we go along.

Talking of books, there is a hand-picked and very eclectic recommended reading list on page 393.

Quick-fix Treat

Shiatsu Face Massage I dropped ten years when I first had this incredible treatment. At that time, I worked in an office, and for the entire working week I had other 30-something women coming up to me and saying, 'You look different. What have you done?' To find a practitioner in your area, call the Shiatsu Society of the UK on 01788 555051.

Supplements

You will never persuade two natural health 'experts' to agree on the exact daily dosage of any single vitamin or mineral that a child should be given. What the supplement makers do is consult with a range of technical experts before deciding on the key doses. Even then, some people will talk about the now abandoned Recommended Daily Allowance (or Dose) (RDA) while others will refer to the more current Reference Nutrient Intake (RNI). Real stalwarts will disregard both these standards and talk, instead, of the importance of the Optimum Nutrition Intake (ONI). The theory here is that the RDAs and RNIs are the amount of a vitamin and mineral you need to prevent illness whereas the ONIs, which are much higher, are the therapeutic dosages that will promote optimum health, strength, resistance to disease and wellness.

The current RNI for vitamin C in the UK, for instance, is just 60mg. The adult ONI for this important vitamin is 1000mg or 1g a day but many of the practitioners I know take twice this amount. (Adults must stay under 2g a day to avoid side effects which can include stomach upset.)

You also need to remember that dosages, even when experts do agree, can never be set in stone because the body's nutrient requirements will vary depending on many internal and external factors, including age, sex, amount of physical activity, climate, season, stress levels, puberty, depression and coping mechanisms, all of which affect the well-being of the body and mind. So, while you can follow guidelines which say a four-year-old needs 45mg of vitamin C daily and a fifteen-year-old male needs 200mg, nobody is going to tell you how much they need when the family is in the throes of a stressful divorce or when they are fighting off a nasty flu virus.

Supplementing Your Child's Diet

In a perfect world, children would get all the nutrients they need from a healthy and balanced diet, but we don't live in a perfect world. So here is a guide compiled by American natural health practitioners to the nutrients that are important, what they do, the tell-tale signs of a deficiency and how dosages need to be increased with age. The dosages here are not therapeutic but are the recommended daily intake designed to maintain good health. The best source of all these nutrients is always from a varied and nutritious diet, but one of the simplest ways to make sure your child gets all this and more is to give them a daily multisupplement from one of the reputable manufacturers (see Which brand to buy, page 94), who will have done your homework for you.

Make sure the brand you are using does not include preservatives, additives or artificial sweeteners (see page 44).

Vitamins Guide for Parents

All dosages are for optimum health, not for treating specific ailments. For the latter, consult a qualified health practitioner such as a nutritionist or naturopath. (See contact details, pages 391–2.)

Vitamin A

Also made from betacarotene (and sometimes called that) in supplements and foods, this is one of the important antioxidants. It can protect a growing child from free-radical cell damage.

What it does: Strengthens the body's mucous membranes, and boosts the immune system, stress-busting adrenal glands and the eyes.

How much kids need:

0–12 months:	375mcg*	(125 IU)
1–3 years:	400mcg	(133 IU)
4–6 years:	500mcg	(166 IU)
7–10 years	700mcg	(233 IU)
11 plus, girls:	800mcg	(266 IU)
boys:	1,000mcg	(333 IU)

*mcg = micrograms, but like vitamins D and E, vitamin A is often measured in International Units (IUs).

Signs of vitamin A deficiency: Eye problems, recurrent infections, delayed growth.

Vitamin B1

All the B-complex vitamins are water soluble: the body cannot store them and will flush any excess from the system. That means they need to be replaced daily. B1 is also easily destroyed by cooking.

What it does: Also known as thiamine, this vitamin plays a key role in the breakdown of carbohydrates from food to make energy. It also supports healthy functioning of the heart, muscles and nerves.

How much kids need:

0–12 months:	0.3–0.4mg*
1–3 years:	0.7mg
4–6 years:	0.9mg
7–10 years:	1.0mg
11–14 years, girls:	1.1mg
boys:	1.3mg
15 plus, girls:	1.1mg
boys:	1.5mg

*mg = milligram

Signs of vitamin B1 deficiency: Persistent tiredness, irritability, depression in older kids and trouble remembering things.

Vitamin B2

Also known as riboflavin and the one most often used to enrich kids' breakfast cereals. The body needs more B2 in times of stress.

What it does: Plays a key role in energy production in the cells and is involved in the breakdown of proteins, carbohydrates and fats from food. Helps the body utilize other nutrients and is important for healthy growth, development of the sex organs and healthy skin, hair and nails.

How much kids need:

0–12 months:	0.4–0.5mg*
1–3 years:	0.8mg
4–6 years:	1.1mg
7–10 years:	1.2mg
11–14 years, girls:	1.3mg
boys:	1.5mg
15–18 years, girls:	1.3mg
boys:	1.8mg

*mg = milligram

Signs of vitamin B2 deficiency: Dry skin, red eyes, cracks at the corners of the mouth, depression.

Vitamin B3

Also known as niacin and another of the B vitamins used to 'enrich' breakfast cereals. The body can make its own niacin from the amino acid tryptophan, which also plays a role in regulating mood. Most supplements use niacinamide to minimize the skin flushing and irritation that can otherwise be a common side effect.

What it does: Promotes a healthy digestion and can help relieve gastric disturbances. Supports a healthy nervous system and plays a key role in the production of the sex hormones. Also needed to maintain healthy skin, and will boost energy by helping the body to break down foods. Can also get rid of bad breath.

How much kids need:

    0–12 months: 5–6mg*

    1–3 years: 9mg

    4–6 years: 12mg

    7–10 years: 13mg

    11–14 years, girls: 15mg

                boys: 17mg

    15–18 years, girls: 15mg

                boys: 20mg

    *mg = milligram

Signs of vitamin B3 deficiency: Insomnia, tiredness, irritability, food rages due to blood sugar fluctuations (see Food Rage, page 179).

Vitamin B5

Also known as pantothenic acid, this is one of nature's own stress busters. It works to support the adrenal glands which pump out adrenaline in times of stress. It can be made in the body by the so-called 'friendly' bacteria in the intestines.

What it does: Helps build healthy cells, supports normal growth and promotes a healthy nervous system. Converts fat and sugar to energy, so important for kids stuck on junk-food diets. Needed by the immune system to make antibodies against foreign invaders. Also supports the sinuses and can help the body recover more quickly from surgery.

How much kids need:

    0–12 months: 2–3mg*

    1–3 years: 3mg

    4–6 years: 3–4mg

7–10 years:	4–5mg
11plus:	4–7mg

*mg = milligram

Signs of vitamin B5 deficiency: Fluctuating blood sugar levels leading to food rages, plus skin complaints. Also, a deficiency in any one of the B vitamins usually means a deficiency in the others too.

Vitamin B6

Also known as pyridoxine, this vitamin is actually made up of three different substances – pyridoxine, pyridoxinal and pyridoxamine – which function together in the body. It is needed to produce hydrochloric acid, which breaks down food in the stomach, and to make DNA.

What it does: The body must have vitamin B6 to produce both antibodies and red blood cells. It breaks down foods to produce energy and helps keep both the digestive and nervous systems healthy. It is also a natural diuretic and so can help prevent bloating caused by water retention. Teens taking the contraceptive pill need increased amounts of B6.

How much kids need:

0–12 months:		0.3–0.6mg*
1–3 years:		1.0mg
4–6 years:		1.1mg
7–10 years:		1.4mg
11–14 years,	girls:	1.4mg
	boys:	1.7mg
15–18 years,	girls:	1.5mg
	boys:	2.0mg

*mg = milligram

Signs of vitamin B6 deficiency: Premenstrual tension (PMT), anaemia, dermatitis, irritability, depression.

Vitamin B12

Also known as cobalamin – the red vitamin – since the body uses it to make and regenerate red blood cells. This is the only vitamin that also contains essential mineral elements. Absorption through the stomach is poor but can be improved when it is combined with calcium (see sections on Synergy, pages 88 and 176).

What it does: Promotes growth and a better appetite in children. Increases energy levels and improves concentration, memory and balance, making it among those nutrients helpful in managing conditions such as ADHD, ADD, dyslexia and dyspraxia (see page 22). Relieves irritability and helps the body use folic acid (see page 72).

How much kids need:

0–12 months:	0.3–0.5mcg*
1–3 years:	0.7mcg
4–6 years:	1.0mcg
7–10 years:	1.4mcg
11 plus:	2.0mcg

*mcg = micrograms

Signs of vitamin B12 deficiency: Pernicious anaemia, irritability, poor coordination. Since the best food source is meat, parents of vegetarians need to take extra care that children get enough vitamin B12. Fish, eggs and dairy products are good alternative food sources for pescarians (people who eat fish but not meat).

Biotin

Also called vitamin H or co-enzyme R, biotin is usually included in most multisupplements and B-complex formulations.

What it does: Relieves eczema and dermatitis and helps keep skin healthy. Plays a role in maintaining healthy hair, sweat glands, nerves and bone marrow. Also, essential for fat metabolism.

How much kids need:

0–12 months:	10–15mcg*
1–3 years:	20mcg
4–6 years:	25mcg
7–10 years:	30mcg
11 plus:	30–100mcg

*mcg = micrograms

Signs of biotin deficiency: Eczema, dermatitis, chronic fatigue, muscle cramps, high cholesterol levels.

Folic acid

Not just for pregnant mums, folic acid is essential for the healthy division of cells and the utilization of sugar and amino acids (used to make proteins) in food but it is easily destroyed by heat and even by storage for long periods at room temperature.

What it does: Can help boost appetite during convalescence from surgery or sickness, plays a role in the production of red blood cells, promotes healthy skin and hair, keeps the nervous system balanced and lowers levels of homocysteine – a by-product of the metabolism of protein that is a 40-times better indicator of the risk of heart disease than cholesterol levels.

How much kids need:

0–12 months:	25–35mcg*
1–3 years:	50mcg
4–6 years:	75mcg
7–10 years:	100mcg
11–14 years:	150mcg
15–18 years, girls:	180mcg
boys:	200mcg

*mcg = micrograms

Signs of folic acid deficiency: Anaemia, digestive disorders, fatigue, skin problems.

Vitamin C

Recent reports suggesting a link between high doses of vitamin C and DNA damage in test-tube trials should be treated with some scepticism. Even the scientists said don't treat this as fact. Thousands of research papers show the many proven benefits of vitamin C. Don't let scare-mongering news headlines or bulletins put you off. The best way to take vitamin C (also known as ascorbic acid) is combined with one of the bioflavonoids such as quercetin, rosehip (which is an excellent natural source of vitamin C too) or rutin (see Synergy, pages 88 and 176).

What it does: What doesn't it do? Speeds up wound healing and will accelerate tissue repair after surgery; acts as a natural laxative; prevents many bacterial and viral infections, and boosts the immune system to fight off coughs and colds. Reduces histamine production during an

Five-star Tip

I use Solgar's Superstrength Rosehip C (£11.85 for 90 tablets) which provides 1,500mg daily to fight off stress. Simply crush the tablet and split into two or three equal doses to take throughout the day yourself. When their immune system is under attack, I give the kids the lower strength chewable version, which provides 300mg daily and which costs £6.79 for 100 tablets. Again, crush and split the dosage. To find your local stockist, call 01442 890355. Adult doses higher than 2g can cause stomach upsets.

allergic attack (see Hay Fever, page 338). Crucial for the healthy growth of teeth, bones, ligaments, gums and blood vessels. Supports the adrenal glands to help the body better cope with stress. Boosts the absorption of iron from the digestive tract by up to 30 per cent, lowers blood cholesterol levels and plays a role in the production of neurotransmitters (chemical messengers) in the brain.

How much kids need:

0–12 months:	30–35mg*
1–3 years:	40mg
4–10 years:	45mg
11–14 years:	50mg**
15–18 years:	60mg**

*mg = milligrams
**Cigarette smoking wipes an estimated 25–35mg vitamin C out of the body every day so teen smokers and kids exposed to second-hand smoke may need increased doses.

Signs of vitamin C deficiency: Scurvy is the best-known vitamin C deficiency disease but is, of course, not a serious risk to most western children living above the poverty line; bleeding gums, persistent allergies and recurring infections would all suggest a need for more vitamin C in the diet or through supplementation. Most vegetables and fruits are an excellent source – kiwi, for instance, is even higher in vitamin C than oranges – but this nutrient is easily destroyed by heat, light, oxygen, smoking and water, making supplementation less of a hit-or-miss affair.

Vitamin D

The sunshine vitamin that is not really a vitamin at all but a hormone. Sunlight triggers the body to make its own vitamin D so try to let the kids spend at least twenty minutes outdoors each day. That said, in the UK we get light of the right wavelength to do this only between April and October, making supplementation a good idea during the winter.

What it does: Crucial for strong bones and healthy teeth – the body cannot absorb calcium, phosphorus, magnesium or zinc properly without it – vitamin D also keeps the immune system strong. It can help relieve conjunctivitis (see page 334) and helps the body assimilate vitamin A.

How much kids need:

0–6 months:	7.5mcg* (300 IU)
6 months to 18 years:	10mcg (400 IU)

*mcg = micrograms, but like vitamins A and E, vitamin D is often measured in International Units (IUs).

Signs of vitamin D deficiency: Severe tooth decay, rickets and other bone and dental problems.

Vitamin E

Don't be misled by the name – this is not a single vitamin at all but a group of eight different but related molecules that subdivide again into two categories called tocopherols and tocotrienols. Of all eight molecules, the most potent is the d-alpha-tocopherol form, so read the label closely and check this is the version you are using. Dl-alpha-tocopherol is a far less potent synthetic version which will be cheaper but less effective.

What it does: An active antioxidant itself, vitamin E also enhances the action of tissue-protecting vitamin A in the body. It is essential for normal cell structure and is so effective for tissue healing that you can reduce long-term scarring by massaging vitamin E oil onto the affected area once the wound has healed. Vitamin E also plays a key role in the formation of red blood cells.

How much kids need:
  0–12 months: 3–4mg* (3–4 IU)
  1–3 years: 6mg (6 IU)
  4–10 years: 7mg (7 IU)
  11 plus, girls: 8mg (8 IU)
        boys: 10mg (10 IU)

  *mg = milligrams, but like vitamins A and D, vitamin E is often
  measured in International Units (IUs).

Signs of vitamin E deficiency: The single biggest sign of a vitamin E deficiency is dry skin.

Vitamin K

This is the jab all newborns get because they are deficient in this vitamin. Again, it is not a single vitamin but a trio: K1, K2 and K3 (the first two the body can make, K3 is synthetic). It can help increase resistance to infection in children but since it is made by bacteria in the gut, it is also destroyed by the antibiotics that kill these bacteria off.

What it does: Vitamin K is needed to produce prothrombin, without which the blood will not clot. It is also essential for healthy bones, where it is used to synthesize osteocalcin – the protein in bone tissues on which calcium then crystallizes. It can help reduce heavy menstrual flow and will promote healthy liver functioning.

How much kids need:

0–12 months:	5–10mcg*
1–3 years:	15mcg
4–6 years:	20mcg
7–10 years:	30mcg
11–14 years:	45mcg
15–18 years, girls:	55mcg
boys:	65mcg

*mcg = micrograms

Signs of vitamin K deficiency: Blood-clotting problems. It may also play a role in coeliac disease.

Minerals Guide for Parents

Calcium

Taking the right form (see page 92) is just as important as getting the dosage right. Calcium is one of the two most common mineral deficiencies in dieting teen girls, and it is needed to help metabolize the other one, which is iron.

What it does: Everyone knows you need calcium for strong bones and teeth but did you know it is needed for healthy muscle contraction, nerve transmission, heartbeat, blood-clotting and cell-membrane functioning too? It is also a potent sleep-inducer and will help beat insomnia.

How much kids need:

0–6 months:	400mg*
6 months to 1 year:	600mg
1–10 years:	800mg
11–18 years:	1g**

*mg = milligrams
**g = gram

Signs of calcium deficiency: Muscle cramping, irritability, insomnia and rickets.

- Do not supplement calcium without supplementing magnesium too. See pages 88–9 for synergy.

Magnesium

Alcohol is magnesium's sworn enemy so kids who may be binge-drinking behind your back may be low in this nutrient.

What it does: Crucial for energy production, magnesium (as well as vitamin C and calcium) plays a key role in the metabolism of blood sugars. It is involved in the formation of the genetic materials DNA and RNA and can help lift mood in youngsters suffering from depression or chronic fatigue (see pages 49 and 54).

How much kids need:

0–6 months:	40mg*
6 months to 1 year:	60mg
1–3 years:	80mg
4–6 years:	120mg
7–10 years:	170mg
11–14 years, girls:	280mg**
boys:	270mg
15–18 years, girls:	300mg
boys:	400mg

*mg = milligrams
**This higher dose reflects the loss of this mineral during early menstruation in pubescent girls.

Signs of magnesium deficiency: Hyperactivity (see page 22), constipation, PMT, chronic fatigue, muscle cramps, depression, irritability and nervousness.

Phosphorus

Playing key roles in growth and tissue repair, phosphorus is present in every single cell in the body but cannot be properly used without vitamin D and calcium.

What it does: Needed for normal bones and teeth, phosphorus also helps maintain a healthy heartbeat. It provides energy by metabolizing fats and carbohydrates, is involved in kidney and nerve functioning and helps the body to better use other vitamins.

How much kids need:

0–6 months:	300mg*
6 months to 1 year:	500mg
1–10 years:	800mg
11–14 years:	1,400mg

*mg = milligrams

Signs of phosphorus deficiency: Muscle cramps, dizziness and bone problems.

Potassium

Potassium works with sodium to regulate the body's water balance but levels are lowered by alcohol and sugar.

What it does: As well as helping the body dispose of waste, potassium helps to maintain steady functioning of the heart, nervous system, muscles, kidneys and blood. It can promote clearer thinking by sending oxygen to the brain.

How much kids need:

0–5 months:	500mg*
6–11 months:	700mg
1 year:	1g**
2–5 years:	1.4g
6–9 years:	1.6g
10–18 years:	2g

*mg = milligrams   **g = gram

Signs of potassium deficiency: Muscle and general fatigue; an irregular heartbeat.

Sodium (Salt)

Helps keep calcium and other minerals in the blood soluble but too much can deplete levels of potassium and cause problems. Parents be warned: shop-bought tomato ketchup is high in salt.

What it does: Essential for normal growth, sodium helps maintain normal fluid levels and works with potassium to regulate the heartbeat. It is also important for healthy muscles and works in the body to support the blood and lymphatic systems.

How much kids need:

0–5 months:	120mg*
6–11 months:	200mg
1 year:	225mg
2–5 years:	300mg
6–9 years:	400mg
10–18 years:	500mg

*mg = milligrams

Signs of sodium deficiency: Although deficiency is rare, fainting, an adverse reaction to heat, and muscle cramps are all signs.

*****

Five-star Tip

If you need to supplement salt intake, which would be unusual, use kelp seaweed, which is a safe and nutritious source.

Quick-fix Treat

Germanium Bath Balls If I took just one product from my bathroom cupboard to survive life with a dynamic five-year-old it would be my germanium bath oil balls. Found naturally in the water at Lourdes and in the energy-boosting herb ginseng, germanium is a semi-crystalline material which literally emits light or photons, giving it a deeply spiritual quality. Twelve bath oil capsules cost £11.90 from Higher Nature (01435 882880). Drop two into a deep bath, soak for twenty minutes and afterwards rest quietly under a blanket for ten minutes before rejoining the outside world.

Trace Elements Guide for Parents

Chromium

Works with insulin in the metabolism of sugar and so is often prescribed by nutritional therapists to help control blood-sugar fluctuations in adult-onset (Type II) diabetes.

What it does: Aids growth by helping to transport protein to where it is needed. Also plays a key role in healthy circulation.

How much kids need:

0–6 months:	10–40mcg*
6 months to 1 year:	20–60mcg
1–3 years:	20–80mcg
4–6 years:	30–120mcg
7–18 years:	50–200mcg

*mcg = micrograms

Signs of chromium deficiency: High cholesterol levels and blood-sugar fluctuations.

Cobalt

This mineral is actually part of vitamin B12 (see page 71) which is known as the 'red vitamin' because it plays such a key role in the production of red blood cells.

What it does: Ensures the healthy functioning of red blood cells.

How much kids need: No RNI or minimum amount has been listed and, in any event, cobalt must be sourced from food.

Signs of cobalt deficiency: Nausea, weakness, pernicious anaemia, loss of appetite, bleeding gums. Milk and meat are the best food sources so strict vegetarians may be at risk of deficiency. Spinach and cabbage are alternatives.

Copper

Utilized in bone formation, copper is also involved in hair and skin colour.

What it does: Copper is crucial for all the body's healing processes but also plays a role in mood. The body needs it to convert iron to haemoglobin – that part of the red blood cells that transports oxygen around the body – and it is crucial for the utilization of vitamin C (see Synergy, page 88).

How much kids need:

0–12 months:	0.4–0.7mg*
1–3 years:	0.7–1.0mg
4–6 years:	1.0–1.5mg
7–10 years:	1.0–2.0mg
11–18 years:	1.5–2.5mg

*mg = milligrams

Signs of copper deficiency: Anaemia, inflammation, recurring infections (because vitamin C cannot do its job without copper).

Iron

Haemoglobin, which accounts for most of the iron in the body, is recycled and reutilized as blood cells are replaced every 120 days. You also need iron to properly metabolize the stress-busting B vitamins.

What it does: Supports growth and development in children. Plays a key role in the production of haemoglobin, and myoglobin which is the red pigment in muscles. Helps build resistance to disease.

How much kids need:

0–6 months: 6mg*

6 months to 10 years: 10mg

11–18 years, girls: 15mg**

           boys: 12mg

*mg = milligrams

**Once menstruating, females lose twice as much iron as males over the course of a month.

Signs of iron deficiency: Tiredness, anaemia, inability to cope with the cold, slower learning skills. The phosphoproteins in eggs reduce iron availability in the body.

Selenium

The new kid on the block, selenium has only just been given an adult RNI yet there is so much interest in it that it is the first ever supplement to be put under the microscope by conventional cancer charities in the UK, who are now interested in its cancer-preventing properties.

What it does: One of the antioxidant big-hitters (see page 182 for HealthClub Bouncers), selenium helps protect the tissues from free-radical damage. It is important for the healthy functioning of the cell membranes, which determine what comes in and out of the cells, and supports pancreatic functioning. It can also help get rid of dandruff.

How much kids need:

0–12 months: 10–15mcg*

1–6 years: 20mcg

7–10 years: 30mcg

| 11–14 years: | 40–45mcg |
| 15–18 years: | 50mcg |

*mcg = micrograms

Signs of selenium deficiency: Skin problems and a dry flaky scalp. Older males may need more selenium than females the same age since selenium is lost in the semen.

Silicon

Also called silica, this nutrient supports the thymus gland which controls metabolism, and works with calcium to make strong bones.

What it does: Key to healthy bone formation, silicon also supports the skin, major blood vessels, connective tissue in the body and thymus gland. It also promotes healthy hair, skin and nails.

How much kids need: No official RNI has been established yet.

Signs of silicon deficiency: Muscle cramps, irritability, poor skin tone, bone problems and insomnia.

Zinc

Although present in all the body's tissues and crucial to numerous body functions – from immune support to protein synthesis – most of the zinc in food is lost in processing.

What it does: Plays a role in energy production, speeds up wound healing, helps the body use the stress-busting B vitamins, regulates the male hormone, testosterone, helps the body break down alcohol, helps maintain the body's acid/alkaline balance (see FoodMates, page 176), works to regulate the production of oil by the skin and is essential for healthy taste buds.

How much kids need:

0–12 months:	5mg*
1–10 years:	10mg
11–18 years, girls:	12mg
boys:	15mg

*mg = milligrams

Signs of zinc deficiency: White flecks on the fingernails, menstrual problems, acne, recurring infections, slow wound healing, stretch marks on the skin, loss of sense of taste or smell.

Quick-fix Treat

Get a Herbal High Most people get addicted to the energy hit a cup of coffee gives them without even realizing they have a problem. If you don't believe me, give up coffee for a week and see how, for the first two days, you feel jittery, get a headache and feel miserable. Wean yourself off coffee, which also interferes with the absorption of other nutrients, especially iron and potassium, using this clever herbal substitute. Herbal Café does contain some caffeine, but only 2mg per dose, which is a massive reduction compared with the 50mg of caffeine in a normal cup of coffee. It also contains the herb Ginkgo biloba which works in the body to enhance memory and keep the mind clear – just like coffee. To get the same energizing hit – a coffee boost without the caffeine – take 2ml (60 drops) dissolved in water or fruit juice. Herbal Café costs £16.95 for 30ml from Revital (0800 252875)

Supplement Synergy – Think Dominoes

We shall see in the Food Talk section of this book (pages 155–234) how the different nutrients in different foods can work with or against each other in the body, and this same idea of synergy is even more important if you plan to give your child supplements. Taking an extra dose of one vitamin, for example, can lower levels of another. Falling short of a specific mineral can prevent the absorption of another, seemingly unrelated one. And too high a dose of a single vitamin or mineral can, ironically, produce the same symptoms as a deficiency in another nutrient. In other words, there is a kind of nutritional domino effect.

We shall see in Food Talk how vitamin C always works best in the presence of the bioflavonoids that give fruit and vegetables their colourings. Vitamin C and copper are synergistic too. Give your child too much vitamin C and you will unwittingly lower copper levels in the body. Without copper, children cannot absorb iron supplies in the diet, which then affects the production of red blood cells, increasing the risk of anaemia.

The very best example of synergy is that of the B vitamins. They are all synergistic with each other and all more potent when used together. Known as nature's own stress-busters, they share many of the same characteristics, including the fact that they are water soluble, which means any excess is not stored in the body but excreted. This means they must be replenished daily.

At-a-Glance Supplement Synergy Table

- **Vitamin A** can help prevent teen acne and protect against cancer in later life but it needs choline, a nutrient the body uses to make brain chemicals (see Bulging Brains, page 237), essential fatty acids, zinc and vitamins C, D and E as well.

- **Vitamin B complex** provides all the anti-stress B vitamins, which also help with digestion, but you also need to supplement calcium, plus vitamins C and E.
- **Vitamin B6** can help relieve PMT but it needs potassium, all the B vitamins in a B complex and vitamin C too.
- **Vitamin C** can protect against the early signs of heart disease, boost immunity and speed up wound healing, but not without bioflavonoids, calcium and magnesium.
- **Vitamin D** is important for growing strong bones but also needs calcium, choline, essential fatty acids, phosphorus and the antioxidant vitamins A and C.
- The **essential fatty acids** (EFAs) are important for energy and brain health but need the antioxidant vitamins A, C, E and the 'sunshine' vitamin D (which is actually a hormone).
- **Magnesium** is essential for nerves and muscles but wiped out by stress. It is the second most common deficiency in post-puberty females. You cannot rebuild levels without calcium, phosphorus, potassium, vitamins B6, C and D.
- **Calcium** is crucial for strong bones but no good without vitamins A, C, D and F plus boron, essential fatty acids, lysine, magnesium, manganese, ipiflavone and phosphorus.

Quick-fix Treat

Kissing Lips Did you know you can ingest up to 60lb (nearly 30kg) of lipstick in a lifetime, or that most of those on sale contain toxic metals such as aluminium and lead? Switch now, and make sure your teen daughter at least starts with one of Living Nature's wild honey lipsticks, which are free from additives and synthetic dyes. Coloured using natural pigments, even the names make you feel warm and better about life – choose from Morning Sun, Pale Moon, Warm Sea, Sunny Day or Laughter. Each lipstick costs £9.75. Mail-order on 01489 566 144.

How to Take Supplements

Giving your children vitamins and mineral supplements should be as simple as identifying which ones they need, working out the correct dosage and then tricking them into swallowing them. In fact, walking into most old-fashioned health stores could not be more confusing. You will be bombarded by hundreds of different supplements and even the exact same thing available in dozens of different forms – all claiming to be the best-ever since sliced bread. You may stand in a daze in front of shelves groaning with capsules, tablets, tinctures, creams, dried herbs, powdered extracts, nasal gels, sublingual lozenges and herbal teas, trying to work out which one to buy. You may even decide it is all too taxing and walk straight out again.

Thankfully, some simple guidelines can help demystify the world of supplements and also ensure your child gets maximum benefits from those supplements you do buy. Here they are.

Buy veggie capsules where you can

Stephen Terrass, natural health expert and former technical director of upmarket brand leader Solgar Vitamins, is adamant that once your nutrients are mixed with food in the stomach, there is no significant difference in the absorption times between capsules, powders or pills – as long as you are buying a brand made by a reputable manufacturer who will have complied with strict disintegration and dissolution requirements. The reason capsules come out on top is that they are easier to digest. But watch out for those made from gelatin – a slaughterhouse by-product. To avoid it, look for brands which say 'veggie capsules' on the label. Powdered and liquid forms may look more appealing but these products have frequently – and especially if they are targeted at kids – been adulterated with artificial sweeteners and other chemicals to improve the taste and smell, so check the label.

Vitamin C

If you want to give your child vitamin C, decide on the dosage and then eke it out over the day. Give one third at breakfast, one third at lunch and the last third at supper. Why? Because the body cannot store vitamin C, which is water soluble, so any excess will leave the body in the urine in under two hours.

B vitamins

These work best when taken all together, so instead of buying single vitamins, buy a good B complex. Known as nature's own stress-busters, these vitamins, like vitamin C, are water soluble, so the same split-dosage rules apply. Look closely at any multi-supplements you are considering and you will see that vitamin C and the B vitamins are the dominant nutrients, so again, don't give one big dose but split it into three equal doses spread over the day. The B vitamins play a crucial role in the manufacture of energy from the food in your diet so it makes sense to give them to your kids at mealtimes. This is not only easier on the stomach, it also recognizes the often overlooked fact that any nutrients we swallow in supplement form will, eventually, interact with the nutrients in food.

Vitamins A, E and D

These are the fat-soluble vitamins which you need to give with food to facilitate their absorption in the body. Also, look for the natural – as opposed to the synthetic – forms, which are easier to absorb. A decade ago, researchers reported that the natural form of vitamin E from soybean oil and wheatgerm, for example, was 36 per cent more active than the synthetic version. Recent research now amends this figure to show the natural form is 100 per cent more active than the artificial one. Once opened, keep the fat-soluble nutrients in the fridge to prevent oxidation.

Calcium

You already knew this mineral was important for strong bones and teeth and now you also know it plays a role in blood-clotting, muscle contraction and proper nerve functioning too. Calcium is a common deficiency in girls, especially those who have started yo-yo dieting. If you decide on supplementation, avoid the cheaper forms including calcium dolomite and calcium carbonate. Invest instead in the more expensive calcium glycenate, or, if this is too pricey, calcium glycinate. This is important because research has shown how women absorb just a fifth of the calcium in the cheaper calcium dolomite supplement but almost half the calcium in a calcium glycinate product. In other words, you get what you pay for.

Hidden sweeteners

Look for supplements that are free from artificial sweeteners (for the long list of names given to the different forms of sweetener see page 45) and other preservatives, including yeast.

Timing

Minerals are best given at the start of a meal and in liquid form because this most closely resembles how they would be sourced in the diet. In contrast, give vitamins at the end of a meal. If you are using a combined vitamin and mineral formulation, give this at the end of the meal too.

Packaging and price

Supplements imported from the US are around 25 per cent more expensive than those manufactured in Europe, reflecting the cost of import duties. On the other hand, a big American manufacturer has the buying power to bulk-buy the active ingredient at a more competitive rate than a smaller European one, which helps close the price gap. Fads and fashions come and go in the supplement market and prices also reflect this. Evening primrose and all the fish oils are always hugely popular; so is glucosamine, which acts to reduce inflammation in the joints. What happens when a supplement becomes fashionable is that some companies take what is called a loss leader and slash their prices to build brand awareness and an increased volume of sales. However, you will still get what you pay for.

Remember, too, there are lots of hidden costs reflected in the price of the more expensive supplements. Those in brown bottles, for example, are better protected from sunlight, which could otherwise cause a deterioration. Plus, these tablets may have gone through a hundred quality tests or more. You will also pay more for products which have more sophisticated delivery systems within the body, such as rapid or timed release, to get the active ingredient to the place you need it. You will pay more, too, if known allergens, such as yeast and sugar, have been excluded from the formulation.

Which brand to buy

Stick with the top names: Solgar (01442 890355), Country Life (020 8614 1411), Higher Nature (01435 882880), Biocare (0121 433 3727), Lamberts (01892 554313). They are all prepared to answer consumer queries about content and manufacturing techniques and although Solgar is now owned by a parent pharmaceutical company that does animal testing, it, like the rest of the companies listed above, does not test its supplements on animals. Where possible, they use veggie capsules and the ethos of all these companies is to promote natural health in a responsible and ethical fashion.

Where to get them

When Tescos carried out a customer survey and said, we've given you organic food, what do you want now?, the answer that came back was unanimous: complementary medicine. The upshot was the setting up of the **NutriCentre@Tescos** and, if not available in any of the two hundred nationwide stores, almost all the supplements recommended here are in the mail-order catalogue. Call 020 7636 0422 for details. The Nutri Centre also has the very best specialist bookshop if you want to learn more about any of the topics covered in this book.

If you like high street shopping, you're in for a treat if you live near any of the **Victoria Health** food shops. For the five London locations and a catalogue, call 0800 413596. For products that may be hard to source, especially those in the A–Z (pages 285–389), I have made specific stockist recommendations.

Revital health stores (0800 252875) run a good mail-order business too and, at the time of going to press, **Boots** was working on a new own-label brand called Alternatives as part of the company's repositioning in well-being and complementary healthcare.

Who to see

The best way to take the guesswork out of supplementation is to consult a qualified nutritionist or naturopath who can run a series of simple tests to determine your child's nutritional levels and to correct any underlying imbalances. To find one in your area, contact the **British Association of Nutritional Therapists** on 0870 606 1284. You will be charged £2 for a referral list. The **British Naturopathic Association** on 01458 840072 holds a list of qualified naturopaths who combine nutrition, herbalism and homeopathy in their treatment programmes.

New Generation Pre- and Probiotics

If probiotics were the first wave of functional foods, then prebiotics will be the next. With a **probiotic**, you use replacement live bacteria to replenish levels of those organisms which live naturally in the gut where they help with digestion and prevent an overgrowth of more harmful organisms. With a **prebiotic,** you go back a nutritional step and selectively feed up the good bacteria that already exist in the digestive tract.

To understand why pre- and probiotics have an important role and enormous potential in nutritional health you have to look at the microbiology of the gut. In a normal, healthy and mature digestive tract, you would expect to find around 3lb (1.5kg) of bacteria. At best, the so-called 'friendly' ones make up a third of this population. At worst, and especially after the prolonged use of antibiotics or years of a diet that is too high in refined foods and sugar, levels of the good bacteria may be so low they are virtually undetectable.

When this happens, it is called **dysbiosis** – a condition that many natural-health practitioners believe lies at the root of more than 70 per cent of all illnesses, including common and chronic complaints such as digestive disorders, acne, food allergies, chronic fatigue and depression.

The advantage of prebiotics over probiotics is that, with many forms of the latter, it is difficult to guarantee the survival of the replacement bacteria after ingestion. The acidic environment of the stomach, for instance, plus the action of bile are lethal to many of the replacement strains. So when you give the kids a pot of live yoghurt – which is rich in good bacteria – you cannot really be sure how much good you are doing. You can't know, for instance, how many live bacteria there are in the pot or how many will reach the colon. And with lots of products, you won't even know what strain of bacterium your child is eating. Live yoghurts do have a place in the healthy diet (unless there is an underlying dairy allergy) but using probiotic supplements takes the guess-work out of rebuilding digestive health.

For maximum effect, give your child a combined probiotic and prebiotic. The latter acts as a food for *only* those strains of bacteria that keep the gut healthy. Clinical trials on humans have already shown this works, using substances called oligo-saccharides as prebiotics. As the name suggests, these substances are sugars derived from plants including garlic, onions, wheat, oats and soybeans. The best known are fructooligosaccharides, usually shortened to FOS.

FOS are not degraded or absorbed in the upper intestinal tract and so can survive the normally hazardous passage through the digestive system to reach the colon. However, it would be a struggle to eat enough of the appropriate plant foods in a normal diet to get any significant effect, which is why you need to consider supplementation.

The reason FOS are so effective is that they only promote levels of the good bifidobacterium strain. This strain is able to thrive on FOS, when other more harmful micro-organisms show no change, because it has a potent enzyme called betafructosidase which can easily break down and digest the FOS molecules.

What to take

A good probiotic supplement will, as we have seen, help replenish levels of good bacteria in the gut. The trouble is, you do not always get what is promised by the label or marketing hype.

Extensive research by UK microbiologist Professor Jeremy Hamilton-Miller of the Royal Free Hospital in London, for example, has shown that many brands fail to contain bacteria either of the strain they promise or in the numbers they claim. In a survey of twenty-nine probiotic products from twenty-six different manufacturers, he found only twelve provided what was stated on the label. His conclusion?

'It is very difficult, if not impossible, for the consumer to know *what they are getting and it was clear, from our research, they were being ripped off.'*

Pre- and Probiotics that Work

- Better known for its fish-oil products, Seven Seas has launched the first multisupplement that combines vitamins, minerals and probiotics. **Multibionta** has been tested by Professor Hamilton-Miller and his team who confirmed it contains exactly what it says on the label. It is also enteric-coated (i.e. covered with a special coating) to protect the ingredients during their passage through the gut. Available from most health retailers, 30 tablets cost £4.49.

- Solgar has announced a new generation probiotic made from two new strains of bacteria: *Lactobacillus acidophilus LA5* and *Bifidobacterium lactus BB12*. The new **Advanced Acidophilus Plus** (60 veggie capsules cost £7.95) for kids over four and the **Advanced 40 Plus Acidophilus** for mums and dads over forty (60 veggie capsules cost £11.19) are both enteric-coated and, unlike probiotic powders, do not need to be refrigerated.

- For younger children (up to 2 years), stick to Solgar's **ABC Dophilus powder** which costs £13.85 for 49.6g and which you do need to keep in the fridge. For local stockists, call 01442 890355.

- The best prebiotic on sale in health stores is still **FOS** which is sold in powdered form too. The sweeter the taste, the higher the purity, so check before you buy. Add to smoothies or breakfast cereals. You can mail-order **FOS powder** (250g costs £6.10) from Revital (0800 252875). Add £1.50 p&p.

- For older kids, **Nutrition Now's Rhino FOS & Acidophilus** combines the pre- and probiotics in an additive-free supplement powder. Mail-order from Victoria Health on 0800 413596 and add 1 teaspoon a day to food or juices. For teens and adults, **PB 8** from the same company contains not two, not four, but eight different strains of good bacteria to aid digestion.

A Guide to Phytomedicine . . . herbs to you and me

A herb is any plant that is valued for its medicinal, culinary or aromatic properties. Not only can you use herbs to relax, soothe and energize the body, but they are also often effective where conventional medicines fail. Antibiotics, for example, cannot eliminate viral infections but many herbs, such as echinacea (pronounced *ek-in-a-shea*), can.

But if you think vitamins and minerals are confusing, try working your way through the minefield that is herbs. On a fact-finding trip to my local (and very small) health store, I found over twenty different formulations that included the best-selling immune-boosting herb echinacea. There were tablets, capsules, powders, tinctures, throat lozenges and sprays. So, how on earth do you work out which one to buy and use?

You really only need to remember two key things:

- Herbal tinctures work fastest but you will not have a clue what dosage of the identified active ingredient you are getting and giving to your child.
- If you want the same benefits you have read about following controlled clinical trials, you will have to take or give the exact same dosage – which means you will need to look for a product offering what is called a standardized extract. What this means is that the manufacturer is promising each tablet or capsule contains at least this specified amount of the active ingredient.

Practitioners who favour tinctures argue that it is better to stay as close to nature as possible and use a preparation that includes all the chemicals in the plant, root or leaf, not just the active ingredient. They also argue those remedies made from wild plants will be more potent because the plant has had more of a struggle to survive. Others say it is better to take a pill, and it is true that in every single clinical trial reporting the proven health benefits of a herb, the researchers were using dried, powdered extracts. This does not mean that herbal tinctures or herbal teas do not work, but if you want exactly the same results, use the same version of the herb (or as close as possible) as those researchers used.

Up to half of all prescription drugs come either directly from plants or are chemical imitations of the pharmacologically active ingredients of a plant. Indeed, our very word 'drug' comes from the German *Droge* which is derived from the word to dry, as in drying herbs. Aspirin, one of the pharmaceutical industry's most successful drugs of all time, is a chemical copy of salicin, an acid derived from the bark of the white willow tree, while digitalis, a drug used to treat heart conditions, copies the active constituents of natural chemicals found in the wild foxglove plant.

What this means is that far from being harmless, herbs can be as powerful as prescription drugs – which is why, of course, they work. It also means they should be treated with the same respect.

Dosages for Kids

Once you have identified the herb or herbs you want to use, take care with the dosages. As well as being very potent, herbs will also affect existing medication so do not mix unless your health practitioner has told you it is safe to do so. Read the adult dosages given on the bottle or pack and follow the advice below:

Under 4 years: Unless you really know what you are doing, seek professional advice (see page 109) before DIY dosing.

4–6 years: Give a quarter of the recommended adult dose.

7–10 years: Give half the recommended adult dose.

11–14 years: Give three-quarters of the recommended adult dose.

15 years plus: Give the adult dose.

Top Ten Herbs for Kids

Alfalfa

One of the best natural sources of protein and high in vitamins A, D, E, B6 and K, as well as calcium, phosphorus, potassium, chlorophyll and iron, alfalfa also provides digestive enzymes to keep your child healthy.

Known as the 'father of all foods', alfalfa is an adaptogen (see page 111) or tonic, which will improve your child's **vitality, well-being** and **overall health**. Sprouted alfalfa is also **rich in fibre** and said to be excellent for **cell detoxification**. If the kids don't like the texture or taste, tuck it into the bottom of a pocket pitta bread packed with hummus, or buy and grind capsules to make a powder you can then sprinkle over food.

Calendula

Herbalists use the flowers, which boast a range of healing properties, from **antifungal** and **anti-inflammatory** activity, to supporting the body's lymphatic waste-disposal system and **promoting the growth of healthy new tissue**. Use a cream to treat nappy rash, insect bites and burns. Make an infusion to **get rid of dandruff** and use internally, as a tincture or tea, to **stimulate digestion** and **boost the immune system's white blood cell activity**.

Chamomile

A wonderful herb for children and another one with many healing properties. Its **antispasmodic action** makes it a good choice for all types of **muscle pain** and **cramp**. Its relaxing qualities make it useful for **relieving digestive disorders** in kids, from colic to constipation and, of course, tummy aches, which in children are a common reaction to emotional upset. Chamomile can help **stop nausea and vomiting.** When used as a steam, the vapours will **break down excess mucus** and so can help clear respiratory infections.

Echinacea

There's a good reason why this has become the best-selling herb both sides of the Atlantic – it works. Once patented and dismissed as 'snake oil' it is, in fact, an excellent overall tonic which can help the body **resist infection-causing viruses and bacteria.** It is traditionally used to purify the blood and so can relieve common **skin complaints including teen acne.** (Purifying the blood simply means sending more blood through the liver for detoxification.) Echinacea has been shown in clinical trials to **stimulate the production of** one of the immune system's major chemicals, **interferon,** and so is now being investigated for the treatment of cancer and herpes too. It works to **cleanse the lymphatic system** and so can also be a useful aid for recovery after conventional drug treatments. Some products now carry a warning saying you cannot use them for children under six. This reflects the terms and conditions of the product's licence, not fact. If you are unsure, use the new Bioforce combination of echinacea and plantago (see Ear Infections, page 327), which has been specially devised for kids.

Fennel

Mix fennel oil with honey and warm water to **relieve a cough.** This mix will also **soothe stomach cramps** and **relieve gas.** Held in high esteem by the ancient Romans, fennel was taken by the men to increase their stamina and courage and by the women to prevent obesity. In fact, fennel tea was prescribed to increase the life span. It is still common practice in India to chew on fennel seeds to help **cleanse the breath** and stimulate digestion after a meal. This herb also acts as a **bronchodilator** and so can help relieve respiratory problems, including bronchitis. Traditionally, it was used to treat colicky babies (see page 313).

Flaxseed

Add flaxseed or linseeds (they are the same thing) to hot cereals to help **relieve constipation**. This works because the herb bulks, softens and moistens the stools to support peristalsis – the wave-like action that moves waste through the colon. Rich in essential fatty acids, especially the omega-3s which are difficult to source from the diet, flaxseed can also help **relieve psoriasis and eczema**. In addition, hospital patients given liquid diets rich in these fatty acids have shown **improved immune function** and more resistance to infections.

Ginger

A powerful **decongestant**, fresh ginger is a must in winter. It will also help **relieve an upset stomach, quell car and seasickness** and warm a cold body. Ginger oil will soothe an ear inflammation, and you can use the fresh juice of crushed ginger root to **soothe minor burns** and **skin inflammations**.

Peppermint

This may not be the world's most exotic plant but peppermint tea is a staple in our household where we use it to support **healthy digestion, relieve nausea** and **bring down a fever**. We make a tea from homegrown leaves but you can now buy capsules too. In older children, it can help **relieve tension headaches** and in babies, it is a **traditional treatment for colic**, the effectiveness of which has now been confirmed by double-blind clinical trials reported in the *Journal of Paediatric Medicine*.

Red clover*

Rich in vitamin A and calcium, the flowering tops of the plant are used to help treat most inflammatory skin complaints, including **eczema** and **psoriasis**, but especially **acne** and **boils**. It also has a mildly sedative action in the body and so was often used to treat **whooping cough** (see page 385). Red clover works to **support the immune system**, making it an excellent herb for children who are convalescing. It has strong **antibiotic properties** and can kill many harmful pathogens, including those causing **tuberculosis (TB)**. To **get rid of fungal infections** such as athlete's foot for good, make a red clover tea and add to the bathwater.
*Do not give red clover supplements to teenage boys.

Slippery elm

Don't you just love the name? Of course, it must have something to do with the gut. You can make a tea with the powdered inner bark or buy ready-made supplements to help **relieve constipation, stomach cramps** and **diarrhoea**. This is thanks to its high mucilage content. You will also find this herb in cough and cold preparations, and you can use it to **soothe an irritated dry throat and rid the body of excess mucus.**

How to use your chosen herbs

Teas/infusions: They're the exact same thing. Use 1–2 teaspoons of the dried herb to 250ml/8fl oz of boiling water. Steep and leave to cool for 5–10 minutes. Strain and drink. Give 1 to 3 cups a day, before meals. Use this method for leaves, stems or flowers, and for roots or bark only if they have been finely powdered. For specific teas, see page 110.

Tinctures: These are fast-acting and allow you easily to mix your own health-promoting combinations. Look for organic products and use as directed on the bottle.

Supplement capsules or tablets: Break open the capsule and smash the tablets to hide the herbal contents in drinks and food.

Steaming: Brilliant for treating respiratory and skin disorders. Put 1 tablespoon of your chosen herb (powder or dried flowers) in a large bowl. Pour 600ml/1 pint of boiling water over the flowers. Taking great care, rig up a makeshift tent using a bath towel to cover your child's head and the bowl and persuade your child to inhale the steam for up to ten minutes or as long as they will sit still.

In the bath: Make a tea (or infusion) with the herb of your choice. Use 1 tablespoon of herb to 600ml/1 pint of water; steep and then strain into the bath.

Topical creams, ointments and washes: You can make your own but when there are so many excellent and relatively inexpensive ones in the shops, why bother? I like Napiers, Weleda and the fabulous new Lotus Emporium range (see page 108 for contact details).

Herbal pillows: These sound fiddly but it doesn't take long (just one episode of *Coronation Street*) to sew a handful of your chosen herb or mix into a small muslin square to place under the pillow at night.

Poultices: One for the serious traditionalists among you. Here, the fresh plant is bruised or crushed to a pulp before being mixed with a 'moistening material' to make a paste to apply to the affected area. You can mix the dried herbs with a little hot water or use a host paste such as flour, bran or cornmeal. Sandwich this paste between layers of sterile, thin cloth or gauze and apply to the wound or affected area.

Compresses: If you've ever placed a warm facecloth over tired eyes then you have already used this technique. Simply soak a sterile towel or cloth in a hot or cold herbal infusion. Wring it out and place gently over the affected area. Repeat several times. If you're in a rush and don't have time to make the tea, you can use this same technique with water to which you have added a few drops of your favourite essential oil (see page 119).

Decoction: This is used to extract the active ingredients from the harder parts of plants – especially the bark, seeds, roots and rhizomes – which only release their chemical after a more prolonged hot-water treatment. Soak 30g of your chosen herb in 500ml/just under 1 pint of cold water for 10 minutes. Pour this mixture into a saucepan, cover and bring to the boil. Lower the heat and simmer for 10–15 minutes. Remove from the heat, keep covered and allow the liquid to sit and cool for another 15 minutes. Strain and drink as a tea, in the same way as an infusion.

Hiding the horrible taste

Most herbs and herbal remedies taste horrid so even when you've chosen the right one, you may still have your work cut out disguising the awful taste. Don't despair, there are lots of ways to sneak the right herbal remedy onto the day's menu with the minimum amount of fuss.

*****
Five-star Tip
Tinctures for Kids
If you cannot find an alcohol-free tincture of the herb of your choice, mix the recommended dosage with 4 tablespoons of very hot water. Leave to cool for 5 minutes, during which time the alcohol will have evaporated away.

I always hide herbs in smoothies and syrups (see page 188). If you don't like the taste or smell then don't imagine your child will. One easy way to sneak bitter-tasting herbal tinctures into the diet is to add the correct dosage to water in an ice-cube mould and freeze it. You can then add these ice cubes to drinks you serve the kids. You can also use this same method to make delicious fruit juice or fruit purée lollipops. Otherwise, buy the herb in capsule or tablet form, crush tablets with a rolling pin or open capsules and sprinkle the resulting powder or oil over food or in sauces and salad dressings.

Which brands to buy

Solgar (01442 890355) has the biggest range of herbal products available in the UK and is the market leader, but other good brands include Country Life (020 8614 1411), Higher Nature (01435 882880), Biocare (0121 433 3727), Bioforce (01294 27734), Biohealth (01634 290115), The Organic Herb Trading Company (01823 401104), Napiers (0131 553 3500), Baldwins (020 7703 5550), Weleda (0115 944 8222) and Herbs of Grace (01638 750140). Lotus Emporium (01225 448011) is another excellent range, especially for teens and mums looking for fabulous herbal beauty products. For teens, I also rate the Kiss My Face American range which describes itself as obsessively natural! For stockists, call 01686 629919.

Who to see

The **British Naturopathic Association**, 01458 840072, holds a list of qualified naturopaths who combine nutrition, herbalism and homeopathy in their treatment programmes. The **National Institute of Medical Herbalists** is on 01392 426022. The **British Herbal Medicine Association** is on 01453 751389.

Dust Off the Teapot!

Making your own herbal teas could not be simpler and if you ever make a pot of loose-leaf tea, you are already doing the same thing. You need to remember to allow the herb of your choice to steep in hot water for 5–10 minutes. Then simply strain and pour.

Many of the healthier teas taste quite planty which kids will hate so sweeten the taste by adding organic maple syrup or honey and find some way to bribe them to drink it all down.

Easy peasy teas

Digestion: Fennel tea stimulates the secretion of digestive enzymes and calms the digestive tract but should be avoided in anyone older with a history of blood clots. Use the seeds for tea.

Insomnia: Chamomile works to relax the body's muscles and prepares the mind for sleep. Make a tea from the flowers. Hops are a good source of the B vitamins which encourage a good night's sleep. Again, use the flowers.

Psoriasis: Red clover is an age-old remedy for skin problems and is a good source of vitamin A which keeps skin healthy. Use the flowers and make an infusion to drink or cleanse the face with. Yellow dock detoxifies the body and reduces inflammation. Make a tea from the root and allow to cool before drinking. (Do not give red clover supplements to teenage boys.)

Diabetes: Bilberries stimulate the production of insulin and lower blood sugars and so make an excellent tea for diabetics and teen girls suffering from a hormonal condition called polycystic ovary syndrome (PCOS) (see page 363), which also adversely affects insulin production. Make a tea from the dried leaves.

Weight loss: A natural diuretic – which means it expels excess fluid from the body – and a natural laxative too, alfalfa can support any concerted effort to lose weight. It prevents water retention, cleanses the whole body, improves the digestion and keeps the intestinal tract healthy. Make a tea from the leaves.

Invest in: A copy of *Herbal Gold* by Madonna Sophia Compton, which is brilliant. Published by Llewellyn Publications in America, I paid £9.99 for my well-thumbed copy.

Mycology Magic

The health superstars of Asian cooking and healing are the mush-rooms that are now classified by modern herbalists and natural healers as **adaptogens** and **immune boosters**. An adaptogen is any herb that makes the body more able to resist infection, cope with stress and deal with environmental and food pollutants – without causing side effects itself. Adaptogens also regulate hormones and blood-sugar levels. In other words, they work on every system to enhance and make it stronger. (Ginseng is a well-known herbal adaptogen. In laboratory trials researchers found that rats who were given this herb not only learned to perform specific tasks faster but made fewer mistakes when doing so.)

These miracle mushrooms also add fantastic nutritional value to any dish. In comparative tests, even those varieties deemed to have less nutritional value rank on a par with carrots and turnips, while those with excellent nutritional properties are matched with meat and milk, making them excellent substitutes for vegetarians and families dealing with food intolerances. They are rich in pro-teins, vitamin C, stress-busting B vitamins and heart-protecting potassium. But to release the full nutritional value, you need to cook them. Here are the **Big Hitters:**

Shiitake: These beefy brown mushrooms, which you can now buy in some supermarkets, have been used by Japanese healers for more than 2,000 years. They stimulate the immune system to produce more **interferon** – a substance that helps the body fight off viral attacks. They also contain a polysaccharide called lentinan which has been shown to slow down the growth of cancer tumours in animals. An excellent source of magnesium (see page 79) and a good source of vitamin D, which kids need to absorb calcium and build strong bones, they unlock their nutritional value when cooked.

Reishi: In Japan 99 per cent of all the wild reishi grow on the barks of old plum trees. However, they are so rare, only a few reishi will be found among a hundred thousand individual trees. Cultivation has increased availability and brought the price down, making this a popular remedy now for the treatment of common childhood disorders, including insomnia, bronchitis, asthma and other allergies.

Cordyceps: Also known as the caterpillar fungus, in ancient China this plant was so rare it was only ever used at the emperor's palace, where it was prepared by stuffing five drams (⅛th of an ounce) of the fungus into the stomach of a dead duck which was then slowly roasted over the fire. Thankfully, you can now buy it in supplement form. It has similar adaptogenic properties to ginseng (see page 111) and so is useful in helping a convalescing child to rebuild strength. It stimulates the production of red and white blood cells and is a powerful antiasthmatic agent. In China, it is used as a lung and kidney tonic and given to treat persistent tiredness, a persistent cough, anaemia and to reduce phlegm and build bone marrow. It can also help regulate menstruation and so could help a teen girl coping with erratic periods.

Coriolus – the new kid on the block: If conventional researchers found a drug or any other agent that could do what this humble herb can do, doctors and others would be shouting the news from the rooftops. As it is, hardly anyone has yet heard of coriolus – a mushroom which has now been shown in UK clinical trials to reverse the cervical cell changes that can otherwise lead to cervical cancers in women.

It's shocking but true that within four years of becoming sexually active (and so this may include your older teen daughter) 80 per cent of women are infected by the human papilloma virus (HPV). The connection between this virus and cervical cancer is undisputed. Cervical cancer is the fifth most common cancer in humans and 90 per cent of cervical carcinomas are believed to be related to an HPV infection. What coriolus has been shown to do is increase the antiviral activity of the body's own natural killer cells, boosting its defences. After some promising early findings, researchers working with Dr Jean Munro at the Breakspear hospital in London are now investigating how coriolus can be used, alongside folic acid, to prevent and even reverse cancerous changes to the cells of the cervix by controlling HPV.

What to take

Triton is a food supplement that combines cordyceps (*Cordyceps sinensis*), reishi (*Ganoderma lucidum*) and shiitake (*Lentinula edodes*) mushrooms, which then work collectively to boost the immune system, increase aerobic performance and counter infection. This supplement contains 166mg of each mushroom and is sold in pots of 90 × 500mg tablets to last for six weeks (£18.95). Three months' supply costs £36. Coriolus costs £18.95 for 90 × 500mg tablets from the same company. Mail-order supplies from the UK specialists Stewart Distribution, on 01273 558112.

If your child dislikes swallowing tablets, crush them and sprinkle over cereals or even mix with the butter in their lunchtime sandwich.

Quick-fix Treat

Zero Balancing Ignore the daft name, which means nothing (literally!). There is no better treatment for rebalancing the body and mind. ZeeBee-ers, as they call themselves, say it's meditation without the mantra, therapy without the talk and massage with your clothes on. The best bit is you just lie on the treatment couch, close your eyes and let the therapist do all the work. Devised by a medical doctor, most ZB practitioners also have serious bodywork backgrounds, especially osteopathy or chiropractic. To find one in your area call the Zero Balancing Association on 01308 420325. Expect to pay from £25 per session.

Homeopathy for Kids

If you sent a homeopathic pill to the lab for analysis, the puzzled scientists would tell you there's almost nothing in it. That's because science cannot yet measure the very essence of the active ingredient which, in homeopathy, is what is said to trigger the body to heal itself.

Homeopathy works by treating like with like. Often, the name of the remedy gives a clue to what you use it for. If, for example, your child suffers from summer hay fever caused by grass and flower pollens, you would give them a homeopathic remedy called Mixed Pollen. If it's Sunday morning and you have a hung-over teen in your house, you might want to serve a remedy called Nux vomica with breakfast.

A homeopathic pill is made up of the active ingredient, diluted down many, many times, and a 'carrier' substance, usually sucrose. The strength or potency of the pill is described with the letter 'c'. For example, the label may read Nux vomica 6c. What you need to remember is that the more a remedy has been diluted, the stronger it is. A remedy that says 200c on the label has been diluted more – and so is more powerful – than a remedy that says 6c. Sometimes you will see an x instead of a c. This denotes an even weaker dilution and so stronger potency.

Homeopaths believe that these remedies capture the very essence, or energy, of the substance they are made from. It is this healing energy that then triggers your own life force to make you well again. According to new research, the idea that an ultra-dilute solution can be as effective, if not more so, than a whopping great dose of a drug may not be as barking as it sounds. When the body is under attack, special white blood cells called basophils release histamine to help counter the onslaught. Once histamine has been released and enough has flooded the tissues, this message is fed back to those cells which then stop histamine production. Scientists set out to prove homeopathy could not work by investigating what would happen if an ultra-dilute solution of histamine was introduced to these same cells. They found the exact same response. In other words, it does work. They did not think the dosage would have been high enough or biologically active enough to make any difference but those basophil cells stopped producing histamine all the same.

The current fashionable theory about how homeopathy works is that although the active ingredient has been diluted down so many times, the water that has been used in this process keeps a memory or 'imprint' of the energy or vibration of the active ingredient. This then does the healing work.

Homeopathy is completely safe. It will not interfere with any medication you are already taking, and it works brilliantly with both young children and animals – proof, say practitioners, that it cannot be 'all in the mind', which is another popular explan-ation for what is going on.

To take or give someone a remedy, you (and they) must avoid touching it, because touching the delicate pill can destroy the potency of the active ingredient. Instead, tip one of the tiny white pills first into the lid of the bottle it came in and then under the tongue, where it will dissolve. It is better to eat nothing for twenty minutes before and after taking a remedy to give it time to work. Once symptoms stop, there is no need to continue with that remedy. If they recur, the remedy can be taken again.

The royal family swears by homeopathy. The reason I like it is that, once you get used to the strange names, it is easy to use and inexpensive. You can keep some of the remedies listed here in your medicine chest at home to treat yourself and your family for the kind of everyday niggles you don't want to bother the doctor with.

If homeopathy appeals to you too, it would be worth seeing a homeopath to have what is called a constitutional diagnosis. Some practitioners train for up to seven years – as long as a doctor – and are highly skilled at diagnosing the right remedy for your type. This is a complicated process and requires an expert but, once done, this may remain your constitutional remedy for life. The idea is that your constitutional remedy helps the body rebuild good health. You can then use the remedies listed below for everyday complaints. That said, these remedies work well anyway and you do not have to have a constitutional remedy to be able to use them successfully.

Everyday Homeopathic Remedies

To decide which remedy best suits your child's problem, read through all the options. A remedy is decided based on many factors, including, for example, what type of pain your child has.

Acne in teenagers: Calc phos if the skin is pale and sweaty, especially good for teenagers. Sulphur if the skin is generally unhealthy, Silica if the skin is sweaty and the spots are slow to clear.
• Give a 6c potency three times a day for 10 days.

Asthma in childhood: Homeopathic immunotherapy has produced excellent clinical results in the treatment of asthma in children. In a French study of 182 children aged between 2 and 8, for example, the homeopathic remedy Poumon histamine was shown to greatly reduce the number of severe asthma attacks.
• Give a 6c potency three times a day until the symptoms pass.

Bruising: Arnica should be used after injuries and accidents. After surgery, Bellis perennis is better.
• Give a 6c potency three times a day for 1–2 days.

Chilblains in winter: Give Cal fluor if the chilblains are cracked and chapped. Also good for circulation and so useful for kids, especially girls, who suffer from Raynaud's disease where poor circulation to the fingers and toes causes pain in cold weather.
- Give a 6x potency three times a day for 10 days.

Constipation: Nux vomica if your child tells you it feels as if he or she hasn't really finished going to the lavatory, Graphites if there is any mucus in the faeces, Bryonia if the stools are hard and dry.
- Give a 6c potency three times a day for 2–3 days, or three doses of a 30c potency remedy, eight hours apart.

Cystitis and other urinary infections: If your child describes a violent, burning sensation, use Cantharis. If it is the last few drops of urine that sting, use Apis.
- Give a 6c potency three times a day for 2–3 days.

Depression/mood swings: When your teen tells you life is no longer worth living, then Aurum is the best homeopathic remedy. If depression is the result of a bereavement or poor exam results, give Nat mur. If you are depressed and exhausted after taking care of others, take Phos ac.
- Give two 30c potency pills, eight hours apart.

Hangovers: If the symptoms include feeling dizzy with a headache that is worse when the head is moved, give Cocculus; if nausea is the main symptom, give Nux vomica.
- Give a 6c potency in 2–3 doses.

Menstrual problems: If period pains start in the small of the back and are accompanied by nausea and cramping, give Caulophyllum; if your daughter complains of throbbing pains with a headache and has a hot, flushed face, give her Belladonna.
- Give a 30c potency three times a day for 2–3 days.

Sleeplessness: If your child complains of feeling too tired to sleep, try Kali phos; for a mind that won't stop racing, offer Coffea, and for fear of nightmares, give Aconite.

• Give one 30c potency pill at bedtime.

Want to learn more?

Homeopathy by Rebecca Wells (Aurum Press, £9.99) helps simplify what can be a complicated field. Rebecca worked for many years with Neal's Yard Remedies in London – a company that was first set up to bring homeopathy to a wider audience. *Homeopathy for Children* by Gabrielle Pinto and Murray Feldman (C.W. Daniel Company) is also excellent (£9.99).

Need a practitioner?

To find out how to get homeopathy on the NHS, contact the **British Homeopathic Association** on 020 7566 7800 and ask for the new patient guide booklet. This organization also keeps a list of doctors who are homeopaths too. To find other qualified homeopaths in your area, contact the **Society of Homeopaths** on 01604 621400. In South Africa, homeopaths do a two-year medical training alongside doctors before specializing. In other words, this is not something you can learn in a weekend course. For best results, find a practitioner who is experienced in dealing with the problem your child is presenting with.

Essential Oils

Essential oils may be simple to use but they are made up of many complex chemicals which give them their healing properties. I never go anywhere without a small bottle of Lavender oil, which few people realize contains over two hundred different chemicals. This is why the same oil can be used for different purposes. I use Lavender, for instance, for relaxation but also as a disinfectant and to wake me up in the mornings.

The important thing to remember is that you should never use essential oils directly on the skin. The most commonly used carrier oils – into which you dilute a few drops of your essential oil – are grapeseed, sweet almond, safflower, soya, sunflower and sesame. (The latter is used in Ayurvedic medicine, see page 133, to draw toxins from the body via massage.)

To benefit from the healing properties of an oil, you need to get it into the body, either through the skin – via massage or by using the oils in the bath – or by inhaling it, which is how vaporizers and oil burners work.

My bathroom cupboard is packed with essential oils but the two I use the most with my young daughter are Mandarin (Tangerine), which is known in France as *the* children's remedy, and Rose. Mandarin works wonderfully to soothe a restless child and, like the gorgeous English Melissa oil (Lemon Balm), will help banish insomnia. Like the flower essences and all plant remedies, essential oils also work on a spiritual level and Mandarin is used to promote happiness and a deep connection to the inner child – that essence of your being that was with you when you were born and which remains with you, unchanged, almost as a witness to your life, until the day you die.

Rose is known as the queen of oils. Said to open the heart chakra and reconnect human love with divine love, it is a wonderful mood-booster. It also works to regulate the menstrual cycle for teens, strengthens the stomach through any emotional upsets and is brilliant for helping to keep all types of skin in good condition.

Safe Dosages for Children

It is not a good idea to use essential oils on children under the age of two, although you can use floral waters or make a bath milk for babies and toddlers by adding 1 drop of either Lavender or Chamomile (both of which are safe for infants) to 20ml of full-fat milk. Add this to their bath.

3–12 months:	1 drop of Lavender or Chamomile oil in 10ml carrier oil or, to make a bath milk, in 20ml full-fat milk.
1–5 years:	2 drops of essential oil, especially Rose or Mandarin, in 10ml of carrier oil.
6–12 years:	half the normal adult dose.
Over 12 years:	adult doses are safe.

In **aromatherapy**, essential oils are first diluted (1–3 drops of the chosen oil in 1 teaspoon of a carrier base oil) and then massaged into the body. Essential oils also work synergistically. Lavender, for example, enhances the already powerful anti-inflammatory properties of Chamomile when you blend the two together.

Working with Essential Oils

Essential oils not only work, they are easy to mix to make your own favourite blends. Until you get the hang of it, try some of my family favourites:

Time out: This downtime bath blend is the perfect antidote to the stresses and strains of twenty-first-century living for kids and parents alike. Add 3 drops of Lavender, 1 drop of Geranium and 1 drop of Mandarin to 5ml of grapeseed oil.

Breathe easy: Eucalyptus is recommended for respiratory problems such as asthma and bronchitis but lots of kids don't like the smell. In any event, I prefer Myrrh, which works as an anti-inflammatory for the bronchial tract. I have a vaporizer* in my daughter's bedroom and use this oil to help relieve her occasional night coughs.

Sleep well: English Melissa, also known as Lemon Balm, is brilliant for treating shock (apply a little of the diluted oil to the temples and pulse points of the wrist) and can also help insomniacs get off to sleep (use an electric vaporizer in the bedroom). Once known as the 'elixir of life', it was even used as a sedative by the Vatican. With strong anti-viral properties, you can use it to treat cold sores and herpes blisters by applying the diluted oil to the affected area. It can also relieve menstrual cramps. Avoid cheap imitations being passed off as the real thing. This is a low-yield plant and you may not always get what you think you're buying. I get mine from **Elixarome Pure Essential Oils** on 01892 833334.

Calm down: Chamomile is a great stress-buster, relieving tension from the mind and muscles. It works well when you have a toddler throwing a tantrum, and can also help relieve stomach problems, eczema and mouth ulcers. It will also help keep you calm when you realize you're actually arguing with a five-year-old. To benefit from its healing properties, use it in your oil burner or vaporizer. To relieve skin complaints and

---

*Oil burners can create a healing atmosphere in the room but in my daughter's room, I use a plug-in, slow-release, electric vaporizer (which can also work as a humidifier), made by Tisserand. It costs £17.99 and is available from most good health stores.

stomach pains, dilute and use as a massage oil. For mouth ulcers, dilute and dab the affected area with a sterile swab.

Pre-menstrual tension (PMT): Deeply relaxing, Clary Sage helps strengthen the body through any kind of convalescence but also works to relieve menstrual muscle cramps. To tackle PMT, you can also use a homemade blend, diluting 8 drops of Geranium, which works to re-balance the hormonal system, with 2 drops of Lavender in 20ml of grapeseed carrier oil. Add this to the bath to soothe away period pains. You can also dilute the oil to massage onto the skin around the stomach and at the lower back.

All worn out: Citronella can boost flagging energy levels and will also act as an insect repellent, making it an excellent remedy to pack for family holidays. Dilute and massage over exposed skin to stop bugs from biting. You can, of course, use the popular Citronella candles to help keep hotel rooms insect-free.

Teen blues: Bergamot is excellent for helping to relieve anxiety, nervous tension and depression. Its combined cooling and refreshing qualities seem to help allay the frustration that lies at the root of a great deal of teen and childhood depression. Add to the bath to lift the mood and enhance relaxation, or use it in your oil burner or vaporizer. It is also very effective against cold sores and chicken pox when diluted and gently dabbed on those sores, and will even keep the family pet off your plants if you burn it next to them.

Teen boils and spots: This is the one time you can use an oil neat. Dab the affected area with Lavender oil which not only has an antibacterial action but which will also accelerate tissue-healing after the infection.

Want to Learn More?

Essential Health – The Complete Aromatherapy Guide by Kolinka Zinovieff is brilliant. It includes a clear and concise guide to the physical, mental and spiritual properties of everyday oils, plus an A–Z guide on how to use them for everyday ailments. The publisher is London Natural Health Press (ISBN: 0952-78250-2) and the author, who is also a cranial therapist, can be contacted on 020 8743 9485. See also the recommended reading list on page 393.

Where to get your oils

Aromatherapy is so popular, you can even buy essential oils and related products in supermarkets, but as with everything in life, you get what you pay for. I buy most of my oils from these two little-known companies whose products stand head and shoulders above so many of the rest:

Devon-based **Touch-Fire Aromatics** run by Peter Neumann specializes in essential oils and incenses from around the world. Even better, you will know exactly what you are getting because the label will tell you. Where possible, the oils are organic, from a single harvest and the country of origin is shown. Contact the company on 01803 762766.

If you want organic oils, check out the high quality **Natural Health Remedies (NHR)** range. These have been created by Kolinka Zinovieff and are excellent. The company also produces organic floral waters, which have similar properties to essential oils but do not need diluting since they have a more gentle action, making them suitable for younger children and babies. Contact this company on 020 8746 0890 or visit the website at www.nhr.kz.

Quick-fix Treat

Stay Zen With a supplement called just that! While Zen was formulated to help avoid panic attacks, it can also help you stay calm whatever the time of the month. It works to boost levels of a neurotransmitter called gamma-aminobutyric acid (GABA), a brain chemical which helps minimize feelings of anxiety, and it contains theanine, an amino acid found naturally in tea and responsible for the soothing benefits of a good brew when you're feeling stressed. Zen costs £19.95 for 60 capsules. Mail-order from the Nutri Centre on 020 7436 0422 and take 1 or 2 capsules daily.

Flower Remedies

Walk into any health store and, again, you'll be bombarded by different types of flower essences too. There are the original Bach flower essences created in England in the 1930s, there are Californian essences made by moonlight and stars, and there are even essences made from prehistoric-looking sea plants. Walk straight by them all and make a beeline instead for the **Australian bush flower remedies** which, in my opinion, should be in every home in the land. Created by Ian White, a trained naturopath and fifth-generation Australian herbalist, the sixty-four different essences in this range have been creating a real buzz here in the UK and when you start to learn more about them, you will see why.

All flower remedies work on the principle that plants have a healing vibration which can help bring the body, mind and spirit back into balance and thus fix the underlying triggers of ill-health. Natural healers would argue that 90 per cent of all sickness stems from emotional and spiritual imbalance and so the key to using flower remedies is to match the healing properties of the plant with both the symptoms and, just as importantly, the emotional triggers of an illness.

The reason the Australian bush flower remedies have captured the collective imagination of healers and practitioners across the world is that they bring the art of flower remedies bang into the twenty-first century and address emotional and social issues – such as sexual abuse and venereal warts – that would have left the more genteel Dr Bach reeling with shock. Parents, too, may not want to think about these things but it has now been shown, for example, that 80 per cent of women will have been infected by the human papilloma virus (HPV) within four years of becoming sexually active, which means your daughter may already be at risk. (I said this earlier, but it's worth emphasizing.)

The bush flower remedies work on a spiritual and emotional level. For example, you may have a child who is asthmatic and you may be all too familiar with the physical or food triggers (see Asthma, page 293), but you may not have stopped to think about the emotional and spiritual factors that may be causing the problem too. For instance, an only child who is living with a single mother who has opted not to embark on any other significant relationship may be suffering from what Ian White describes as 'smother love', where the emotional boundaries between mother and child have become blurred. He explains how this has become increasingly common, where, for example, a mother lives alone with her son who then assumes the role of the man of the house, and how one of his remedies, Little Flannel Flower, can help children who have become old before their time and who may have adult reponsibilities on their young shoulders.

Thus, the combined bush flower treatment for asthma might include not only Crowea, which is effective in relieving the spasms and contractions that are typical of an allergic reaction, but also Little Flannel Flower to counter those feelings of being 'smothered' and unable to breathe, plus Grey Spider Flower to help relieve the terror of an acute asthmatic attack. The idea is not that only 'smothered' children suffer from asthma, but that if you look beyond the physical symptoms, you will find an emotional imbalance that you can also treat.

Taking the Remedies

The Australian bush flower remedies could not be easier to take or give to kids. You can disguise the alcoholic taste (brandy is used as a preservative) by hiding the doses in food. For older children, keep the remedy by the side of the bed so they can take seven drops on waking and seven drops just before sleeping at night. You can also burn the essences in the oil burners you use for essential oils.

Once you start to investigate the bush flower essences, you may think both you and the kids would benefit from taking almost all of them. The key to working out which ones you (and they) actually need is to pinpoint what is going on right now. For example, a child who has issues of abandonment would benefit from taking the Bluebell remedy, but if they are facing tough school exams next week then Isopogen, which works to support memory function, would be a better remedy in the short-term.

If you are tackling underlying issues, give the chosen remedies as directed for two weeks and then review any change in attitude or outlook. For acute problems, give a higher dose of the remedy (10 drops every three or four hours) throughout the day and continue for two to three days.

I agree with Ian White who says of his essences: 'As society changes, new essences come through to meet those changing needs. That does not mean the old essences do not work, but these new ones really do address the real issues now affecting families and their kids.' The other reason I rate this range so highly is that these remedies work fast!

At-a-Glance Guide to Using Bush Flower Remedies

Don't be put off by the unfamiliar names of these plants, which are all native to the Australian bush. As you get to know them, you will love them as much as I do. Remember, you cannot overdose on these remedies, which work at a level 'above' herbs or prescription medicines. They work on our psyche and our energy and vibration. They are completely safe, leaving you free to experiment with what's right for you and your family.

Bush Fuchsia: Works to integrate the left and right hemispheres of the brain and so can help overcome the problems of dyslexia. This remedy also works on the voice and is excellent for kids who stutter. If you have a daughter taking the contraceptive pill, Bush Fuchsia can help re-regulate the hypothalamus gland which will have been affected.

Bush Gardenia: The recommended remedy for truculent and hormonal teens who have trouble communicating their feelings, and for younger kids locked into an unhealthy sibling rivalry.*

Bush Iris: Ex-smokers who have taken this remedy to help clear toxins from the lymphatic system (which drains the body's waste products) report yellow nicotine stains appearing (and eventually fading away again) on the fingers they used to hold their cigarettes in. One woman who had this reaction had not smoked for fifteen years. This is also a good remedy for anyone who has had surgery under a general anaesthetic.

Crowea: The chosen remedy for respiratory disorders, including asthma and bronchitis, but also the remedy to give to kids who worry too much.

Dagger Hakea: The name almost tells you that this is the remedy for anyone bursting with resentment. If you're trying to make a step-family work or help kids get over a divorce, this is the remedy for you. Cleverly, this is one of the ingredients in the new Relationship Combination Essence since it recognizes that much of the trouble between men and women boils down to long-held and difficult to resolve old resentments.

Fringed Violet: Protects the body, mind and soul from emotional and physical shock. Use for acute reactions but also to release shock patterns the body has held on to after, say, surgery, a car crash or an emotional trauma. This is also the remedy for newborns (yes, it is safe for infants) who need their auras or etheric body protecting from outside influences.

*See what I mean, these are the remedies for the kinds of family issues real mums and dads actually have to cope with and worry about!

Grey Spider Flower: Use this remedy to allay the terror of an asthmatic or allergic attack or a violent sickness. It is also the recommended remedy for children suffering from night terrors and nightmares.

Isopogen: Helps kids through exam stresses and learning or behavioural problems – and has to be a better bet than Ritalin, which is similar in its chemical properties to cocaine. (See Difficult Behaviours and Learning Problems, pages 22–7).

Mulla Mulla: The remedy for sunburn, and one to keep in the family medicine chest for emergency first aid and treating all kinds of burns. This remedy can also support anyone undergoing conventional cancer radiation treatments.

Warratah: Helps clear deep-rooted patterns of fear so it can be useful at exam time and for helping your child to overcome anxiety and even phobias.

Want to learn more?

Invest in a copy of Ian White's brilliant book, *Australian Bush Flower Essences* (Findhorn Press, £11.95), which explains in detail all the healing properties of the remedies in the Australian bush flower range. Mail-order the book on 01309 690582. Ian is now a regular visitor to the UK where he runs a three-stage training programme which is invaluable for parents and practitioners wanting to dig deeper into the philosophy and practice of the bush flower remedies. For details and to order the combination or individual remedies, contact **Ancient Roots** on 020 8421 9877, fax on 020 8950 7733, or visit the excellent website at www.ancient-roots.com.

Traditional Chinese Medicine (TCM)

Traditional Chinese Medicine or TCM has one thing in common with western medicine – both start with a good look at the state of the tongue. In western medicine the doctor will be looking at the tongue to see if there is a coating, which is a sign of infection. Chinese healers look at the coating too, but take the whole idea of tongue diagnosis much further.

We use our tongue to taste, chew and swallow our food, and in good health it will look pink and fleshy. The surface will be covered by a thin layer of moisture and there will be no cracks or spots. The whole tongue will be a nice, even, symmetrical shape.

Colour changes to the surface can signal underlying health problems. To the TCM practitioner, a very pale pink tongue, for instance, is a sign of 'blood deficiency'. This doesn't mean your teenager's been hobnobbing with vampires all night but that he or she needs 'building up', starting with the blood. And if this is the case with anyone in your family, you need to consider age-appropriate iron supplementation to prevent weakness and anaemia.

Purple-coloured spots on the tongue reveal a sluggish blood flow, while white spots are said to signal a stagnation in chi – the body's invisible but potent energy or life force. ('Chi' is used in Chinese medicine to describe the energy circuits in the body which cannot be seen but which respond to treatment, especially massage, reflexology and acupuncture, or for kids, acupressure. See Hands-on Treatments, pages 136–53).

The tongue is the only internal organ visible from the outside of the body and so, to Chinese healers, it is no less accurate an indicator of what is happening internally than an X-ray. To work out more precisely what is going on inside the body, TCM healers divide the tongue into ten different parts, each of which link to a specific internal organ. A swelling at the tip of the tongue, for instance, indicates a link back to the heart. This doesn't mean anyone is going to have a heart attack or need surgery. It simply indicates there may be a general weakness in this body system compared with other parts, and that the chi or energy here needs rebalancing and strengthening.

Teens be warned: fine cracks to the left of the front portion of the tongue are a tell-tale sign of smoking, and bumps or other disturbances to the middle area of the surface indicate a tendency to suffer digestive problems.

TCM believes that sickness is a reflection of imbalance in the body and that the most important balance is that between the yin and yang – two opposite but complementary forces. Yin is the receptive female energy represented by the moon; yang is the hot, aggressive masculine energy. We all have both these energies and throughout our lives the dynamic between them fluctuates constantly.

TCM practitioners also believe that like all other matter, the human body is made up of five elements – wood, fire, earth, metal and water – and that, again, each element corresponds to a different organ or a different sense, even different emotions. Working out which element is dominant in the patient is another key in TCM diagnosis.

The critical difference between the approach your family doctor will take and that of a TCM healer is that where the doctor will make a diagnosis and treat only the affected part of the body, the TCM practitioner will, in making the diagnosis, consider everything, from diet to mood, that will be having an impact on the health of your child.

Having made the diagnosis, the TCM practitioner will then use a combination of nutritional advice (beetroot, for example, to build the blood), acupuncture or acupressure and complex Chinese herbal remedies to help rebalance the yin and yang and the five elements, and thus relieve or prevent sickness.

So what's very clear is that TCM is not a DIY regimen. For the very best results you need to find a qualified and experienced practitioner who can build up a picture of the health and history of each member of your family and prescribe a tailor-made treatment programme for them when things go wrong.

Where now?

The **Register of Chinese Herbal Medicine** is on 0700 790332. Call for details of qualified and approved TCM practitioners. The **British Acupuncture Council** is on 020 8735 0400. To find a doctor who practises acupuncture, too, call the **British Medical Acupuncture Society** on 01925 730727.

At-a-Glance Guide to the TCM View of the Body

According to TCM, perfect health is only possible when not only the yin and yang but also the five following elements are all balanced in the human body.

The Elements

Fire: Linked with the heart and intestines, the tongue is the sense organ and the blood vessels are the body tissues ruled by this element. Its ruling emotion is joy.

Wood: Controlling the liver and gallbladder, this element also rules the eyes and the tendons that attach muscle to bone. The emotion is anger.

Earth: Ruling the stomach and the spleen, the sense organ is the mouth. It links to muscle and the dominant mood is meditation.

Metal: Controlling the lungs and large intestine, the sense organ is the nose and its body tissues are the skin and hair. The overriding emotion is grief and/or melancholy.

Water: Ruling the kidneys and the bladder, the sense organ is the ear and the body tissue is bone. Fright and fear are the dominant emotions.

Quick-fix Treat

Lift Your Mood All Natural's Orange, Lemon or Lime Mate air mists are made from 100 per cent pure oils and contain no propellants, fluorocarbons or man-made chemicals. They cost £8.95 for 204ml and you can recycle the aluminium cans. Mail-order on 01273 703461 and spray the room to improve everyone's mood!

Ayurveda

A few years ago, few people outside India had even heard the word Ayurveda, let alone been told its meaning or how to pronounce it. It means 'the science of life' and if you are still not sure, the pronunciation is *eye-ur-vee-dah*.

In urban India, there's an Ayurvedic practitioner on every street corner in much the same way we used to have chemists here. Even in the UK, both Tescos supermarket and the Body Shop now sell specially developed Ayurvedic beauty and personal-care products, and you can't get more mainstream than that.

So how does it work?

Like all natural healers, including western naturopaths, Ayurvedic doctors treat the whole body, not just the symptoms of a disease. They rely on a combined approach using aromatherapy, herbal medicine, diet, nutrition, massage, yoga and even astrology to work out what is wrong with someone and how best to treat them.

If you want to split hairs, the Ayurveda that is offered to westerners is a much watered-down version of the real thing. But, unless you relish the idea of enemas, fasting, vomiting and even swallowing dishcloths to cleanse the stomach – all of which are common practices in true Ayurveda – do not complain.

If you or anyone in the family is interested in this form of healing, then check out the new high street and supermarket Ayurvedic ranges that suit your specific 'type'. There are three different energies or types, which are called 'doshas'. Think of these as being a bit like your astrological birthsign. The first is called Vata, which is the air type. Pitta is a fire energy, and Kapha is a heavier earth type. Now all you have to do is work out which one describes you best. (If you're not sure, ask a mate!)

At-a-Glance Guide to Ayurvedic Doshas or Personality and Body Types

Vata: These types are always on the go. Highly creative and imaginative, they're great fun to be with but they can get a bit carried away and all that nervous energy makes them extra prone to stress and exhaustion. If this fits, watch out for the digestive system which is always the first one to give way. Vata types need to eat regular meals and watch for burnout, even at a young age. Golf, yoga and dance are all great ways to chill out and avoid too much stress.

Pitta: The Pitta child is so dynamic and full of passion, it's a case of once met, never forgotten. They love to be the boss but can become overbearing, so watch out for this trait. Encourage the Pitta child to be less competitive and, as he or she gets older, to curb what can be a nasty tongue. Divert some of their competitive intensity by encouraging activities which do not focus on winning – especially swimming, cycling or snowboarding, just for the fun of it.

Kapha: Solid and as reliable as the earth beneath your feet, these types are the most stable of all three doshas. The only trouble is they can be so laid back, especially as they get older, they're in danger of falling over. Kapha types can skate dangerously close to being lethargic and need to make extra sure they keep their energy levels boosted with a healthy diet and some kind of get-up-and-go activity. Encourage running, tennis or climbing if this describes any of your kids.

If you hate the sound of the dosha that best describes any of your children (or even you), don't despair. We're all made up of all three types of energy and in perfect health there is a balance between them. This is what the Ayurvedic doctor tries to achieve using certain foods, herbs and massages. Your type simply describes which energy is the dominant one.

As well as recommending changes to what, when and how to eat (preferably slowly and sitting down), the experienced Ayurvedic practitioner will also introduce the idea of a detox massage. There are lots of different types of Ayurvedic massage but my favourite involves having warm oil gently poured onto the middle of your forehead where your mystical third eye is. After twenty minutes of this, you really do think you've died and gone to heaven, and if you're a stressed-out mum or dad, I can't think of a better treat!

Want to know more?

The Complete Book of Ayurvedic Home Remedies by Vasant Lad is a good introduction. Published by Piatkus, it costs £12.99. To find a qualified practitioner, contact the **Ayurvedic Medical Association UK** on 020 8682 3876.

Hands-on Treatments

When seeking hands-on treatments suitable for kids, you need to take the same if not greater precautions than when finding a practitioner for yourself.

Here are the key rules:

1 Do your homework. Ask about the practitioner's training and accreditation. Complementary medicine is still unregulated and mostly self-policed, which can mean people setting up in practice and charging fees when they have very little real experience. Of course they have to start somewhere, but you do not want your child to be the guinea pig.

2 Make sure the practitioner you choose has previous relevant experience. If you have a specific problem, such as an adverse reaction to the MMR vaccine (see Vaccines, page 5), then find someone who specializes in that area. Similarly, if your child has a digestive disorder, find a naturopath who understands how the gut works and why things can go wrong.

3 Ask around. An enthusiastic recommendation from another pleased mother is the best reference a practitioner can hope for. If you cannot find someone the word-of-mouth way, turn to page 391 for a list of the governing bodies of key organizations.

Acupressure

Acupressure is a superb and very gentle alternative to acupuncture, and since no child in its right mind is going to lie still while 'the nice lady' sticks needles in them, this is the best way to give kids the exact same health benefits. Even better, for general well-being and pain relief, you can learn to do it yourself.

With acupuncture, the needles are inserted at specific points in the body to help rebalance not only the flow of energy – what Chinese healers call chi – through the body, but the underlying energies of specific organs too. (See Traditional Chinese Medicine, page 130.) With acupressure, instead of needles you use the thumb or fingers, applying pressure at the same energy points and with the same goal – to rebalance all those energies.

The best time to work at home with this technique is in the evening, after your child has had a relaxing, warm bath. It is important they stay warm so use blankets and, if it is bedtime, work on the body through their pyjamas. Remember that this is an experience you both need to enjoy so take your time. Reassure your child as you work on his or her body and set the right mood by playing relaxing music in the background and by burning lavender or rose oils, both of which also relax the body.

You need to apply the same pressure to the same points on the left and right sides of the body at the same time, so make sure your child is comfortable and you have enough space to manoeuvre around the body, back and front. If your child is lying down, you may need to ask him or her to turn over.

The pressure you are aiming to achieve is called 'threshold pressure' which means firm but stopping short of painful. Take care not to hurt your child, of course, but try to be firm and gentle. The reason you need some pressure is that you are trying to stimulate this energy point to tonify it, which simply means generating more chi in that part of the body and in the organs it is linked to.

The idea is to apply consistent pressure on both sides for between one and five minutes but at the start, and until you are more experienced, simply apply the pressure for 10 seconds on both points, release for 10 seconds, and reapply. You can repeat this cycle five times before moving on to the next point.

You will soon know if you are applying too much pressure as your child will yelp and instantly draw away from the pain. The best advice is to practise first on yourself and then on another adult before putting your hands on your child. Acupressure can help reinforce the intimacy between you and your child and can be particularly soothing to a child recovering from illness. You will find those acupressure points related to your child's specific complaint will be more tender than other ones you may work on.

To interpret the **Acupressure Map** of energy points that are commonly used with kids on pages 140–1, you need to understand how the points you will be working on are labelled. I know it sounds a little complicated at first but you will soon get the hang of it and discover for yourself just how effective this treatment can be and, even better, how much your child will like and respond to it.

All you need to know is that Chinese healers have mapped out twelve lines called meridians which run along each side of the body. Energy flows along these lines and each pair of meridians (one on each side) corresponds to a specific organ in the body. Each point is named first for the meridian it lies on e.g., the stomach meridian, the lung meridian, the bladder meridian, and then for its position along that line, e.g. Lung 6, meaning the sixth energy point on the lung meridian.

At-a-Glance Guide to Acupressure Points for Common Childhood and Teen Complaints

- To relieve **constipation**, treat **Large Intestine 11** on the arm.
- For **headaches**, treat **Large Intestine 4** at the base of the thumb; this controls the head. Rubbing the muscles that run alongside the spine will also help.
- For **hiccups**, treat **Pericardium 6** on the inside wrist, which will relax the chest.
- For **flu**, treat **Lung 7**, which is also on the inside of the wrist and which will help clear respiratory infections. **Bladder 11, 12, 13** and **14** alongside the spine on the back also clear congestion here.
- **PMT and bad period pains** will be relieved by **Bladder 20** in the mid back and **Bladder 28** in the lower back, both of which relax the nerves of the cramping uterus.
- To treat **nausea** and **vomiting**, work on **Pericardium 6** on the inside wrist, and **Stomach 36** at the knee, which tones the digestive system.
- For **sore throats**, treat **Lung 7** on the inner wrist which will relieve irritation and **Large Intestine 4** at the base of the thumb which can help clear the infection.
- To stop **diarrhoea**, treat **Stomach 36** at the knee.
- Treat a **cold** by working on **Bladder 11, 12, 13** and **14** to rebalance the respiratory system, **Large Intestine 4** to relieve congestion and an accompanying headache, and **Lung 7** to clear infection from the upper respiratory tract.
- For **insomnia**, treat **Bladder 60** at the back of the heel which will bring energy down away from the head and **Pericardium 6** on the inner wrist which relaxes the mind and stops it from racing.

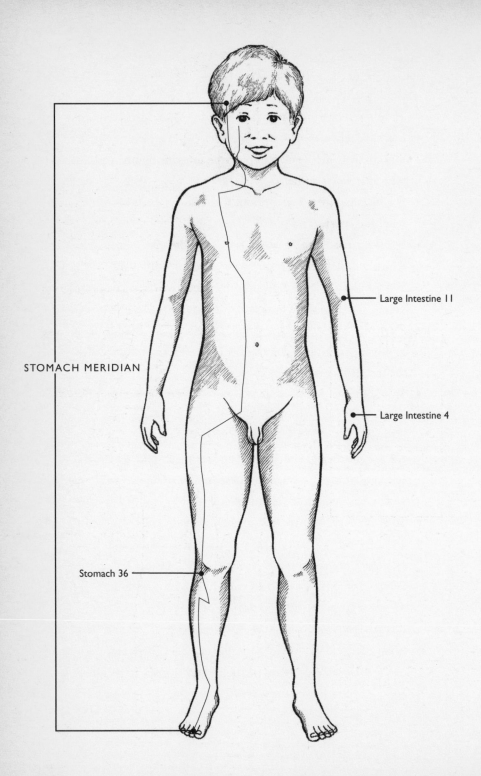

STOMACH MERIDIAN

Large Intestine 11

Large Intestine 4

Stomach 36

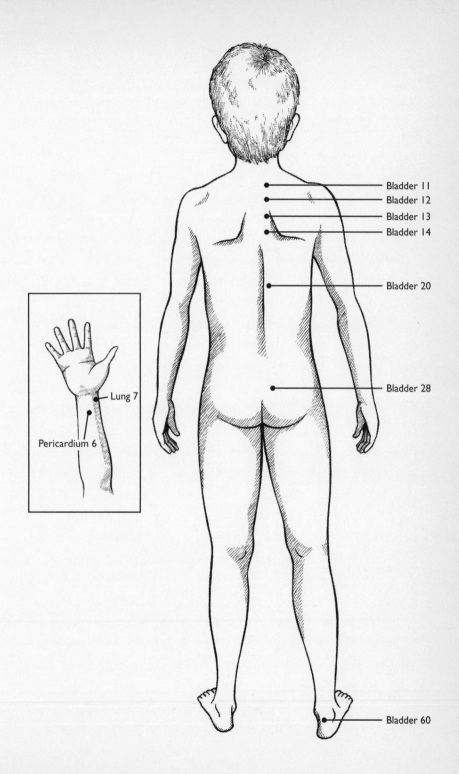

Bladder 11
Bladder 12
Bladder 13
Bladder 14

Bladder 20

Bladder 28

Lung 7

Pericardium 6

Bladder 60

The Bowen Technique

Excellent for treating sporting and other accidental injuries in kids, this is another of those hard-to-explain-how-it-works therapies that has a growing body of good empirical evidence telling us it really does work. Again, it will only be as good as the person practising it, so do your homework and go to the best.

In simple terms, this is another way of manipulating muscles to trigger the body to kick-start its own healing systems to finish the repair job following injury or surgery. During a treatment session, the therapist will run his or her fingers and thumbs across the muscles, tendons and ligaments of the affected area using only very gentle pressure. These movements are like a 'roll' which disturbs the muscle just enough to create an energy surge. The treated area is then left alone to assimilate and react to this disturbance.

Nobody really knows how or why this technique works. One idea is that it triggers a little-known communication system between the body's cells and the brain, which then organizes the repair of damaged tissue or, in the case of tennis elbow, the damaged tendons.

People who have benefited from this treatment say they feel very relaxed afterwards and, although what you will see in those areas where pressure has been applied is an extraordinary red welt-like mark appearing, it is totally painless and completely safe for kids.

This, of course, is not a DIY technique. It attracts a lot of therapists who already have a medical background in, say, nursing or physiotherapy, so you know your child will be in safe hands. There is nobody in the UK currently specializing in treating kids but many therapists treat the whole family and offer the treatment to help maintain good health and to ward off bugs and sickness. There is also good anecdotal evidence it can help children cope with emotional upset and stress, especially around very difficult times, such as bereavement and divorce.

The technique has been used to help children with a long history of bedwetting to stay dry at night, and to help teens recover quickly from musculoskeletal disorders such as tennis elbow. A handful of Bowen therapists also report excellent results with children who have cerebral palsy. The mothers of babies with colic have reported no further symptoms after just one treatment session, and there are also stories of kids with asthma having no further attacks. In other words, there's enough here to check it out!

To find a practitioner in your area – and in the UK, about 80 per cent of Bowen therapists are women, many of whom will have worked on their own kids – contact the **European College of Bowen Studies** in 01373 461873.

Infant Massage

Massage just gives a name to something we all do automatically anyway – notice how you rub your temples when you have a headache and how your child rubs his elbow when he's banged it on a cupboard. It is now widely practised throughout hospitals in the UK and used on kids from newborns to teens. Here are just a few of the health benefits of a relaxing massage: it will strengthen the developing immune system, help flush out toxins, provide sensory stimulation to your baby, and maintain that all-important loving intimacy between the two of you.

Lots of practitioners working in complementary health start out with a massage qualification and the **British Massage Therapy Council** (01772 881063) keeps an up-to-date referral list of trained therapists who specialize in infant massage. That said, it is easy to learn some of the simpler techniques to practise with your baby yourself, and to treat some of those niggling everyday upsets such as trapped wind.

Set the mood using a vaporizer and your favourite essential oil, but to massage a baby or any child under two, use a carrier oil (see Essential Oils, page 119) on its own or gently massage the skin using no oil. Let your own instinct guide your hands and your baby will soon let you know how much it likes it. If you want to help relieve digestive problems or wind, gently massage the lower abdomen in a clockwise direction.

You'll find your child's solar plexus in the middle of the torso, just above the navel. This control centre is rich in nerve endings and, according to Chinese healers and reflexologists, can affect the energy flow to both the abdomen and the brain. Massage this point to soothe an irritable baby, to prevent insomnia in your toddler and to stop a panic attack in older kids and teens.

The Metamorphic Technique

This is one of those hands-on therapies which those of us who swear by like to keep quiet – not least because skilled practitioners are few and far between. If the secret about how brilliant it is ever got out, none of us would ever get an appointment again.

A spin-off from reflexology, the metamorphic technique was first developed in the 1960s to help treat what we would now refer to as autistic children. Good practitioners describe how they simply 'hold' the energy while your child's own life force gets to work to eliminate emotional blocks that might be preventing him or her from reaching their full potential or perhaps causing behavioural problems.

The theory is that from the very moment of conception, traumas are held within the memory of every cell in the body, and until these memories are released an individual cannot make progress. These releases are triggered by a gentle foot, hand and head massage which most children find reassuring. Your child remains dressed throughout a session and will only remove shoes and socks. Most of the children I know who have regular sessions take a favourite video to watch during the treatment and, although not a talk therapy, it is best if parents stay out of the room where their presence may be inhibiting.

To learn more about the metamorphic technique and to find practitioners who are happy to work with children, contact the **Metamorphic Association** on 020 8672 5871 or visit the organization's website: www.metamorphic@britishisles.freeserve.co.uk.

Hand Reflexology

Everyone knows you do reflexology on the feet, but hand reflexology is just as good and even quicker for kids who can't sit still. You can do it any time, any place, and once you know which part of the hand to work on, you can use it to help relieve specific health complaints as well as to bring the body's energy flow back into balance, which is the ultimate aim.

The feet are rich in nerve endings, which is why they are traditionally used by reflexologists to stimulate the flow of energy throughout the body, but whether working on your hands or your feet, what therapists are doing is clearing out energy blockages to prevent or help treat illness. They will also have learnt how the internal organs of the body are mapped out on both the hands and the feet.

The right hand, for instance, mirrors the right side of the body and its organs, including most of the liver. This is a good place to start with a child who has low energy and digestive problems such as constipation. The right hand is also home to the lymph reflex point and another reflex point, between the thumb and index finger, that stimulates the adrenal glands which help the body cope with stress. Stimulate these points (see diagram opposite) by rotating the tip of your index finger in a clockwise direction and pressing down.

No good reflexologist will make any medical claims but this treatment can help alleviate an enormous number of conditions, ranging from skin problems to diarrhoea. It is a wonderful introduction to the powers of natural healing and preventative medicine, and is a fantastic tool for helping your kids to learn to relax, for relieving anxiety and for helping them to cope better with the stresses of everyday life.

*****
Five-star Tip

If you would like to experience and then learn how to practise hand reflexology on your family, contact the **Practitioners' School of Reflexology** and its founder, Andrew James, on 020 8948 2380. The 2-hour treatment, which includes being taught DIY Hand Reflexology, costs £50. A foot reflexology treatment is £40. Hand reflexology, which takes 30 minutes, is £30. There is also a training video which takes you step-by-step through the hand reflexology programme.

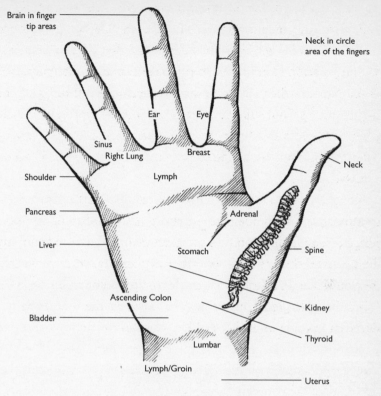

Brain in finger tip areas

Neck in circle area of the fingers

Ear

Eye

Sinus

Right Lung

Breast

Neck

Shoulder

Lymph

Pancreas

Adrenal

Liver

Stomach

Spine

Ascending Colon

Kidney

Bladder

Thyroid

Lumbar

Lymph/Groin

Uterus

Right Hand

At-a-Glance Guide to Easy Hand Reflexology

- To tackle **obesity** and help a child maintain steady weight loss, stimulate the **Thyroid** point, which is just above the wrist.
- To ward off winter **coughs** and **colds** and to re-energize an exhausted child, use the tip of your index finger to rotate the **Lymph** point in a clockwise direction.
- To relieve **teen brain fag** at the end of revision or exams, press the tip ends of the fingers on both hands.

- To treat everyday **digestive disorders**, including constipation, diarrhoea or wind, walk your index and second fingers, caterpillar-style, from the base of your child's little finger over to the base of the index finger. Repeat three or four times on both hands, working your way down towards the base of the thumb.

Yoga for Kids

Yoga teachers and sports scientists working with both primary and secondary schoolchildren are reporting alarming levels of stiffness in a new generation of kids who, thanks to computer games, digital TV, schools with no playgrounds and busy parents who don't exercise either, have little or no body awareness.

The upshot of this is that we are raising a generation which, hampered by tight shoulder girdles, ribcage restrictions and tight hamstrings, finds it uncomfortable to either stand or sit up straight. Next time you see a group of kids together, look at their backs and see if you can detect any hint of abnormal curving of the spine – a condition known as scoliosis. This occurs in only about four per cent of kids aged ten to fourteen (and mostly in girls) but will become more prevalent if you do nothing to help youngsters build the muscular strength and stability needed to support the natural curves of the spine.

Children do yoga naturally. Just watch any group of under-fives at play and watch how they twist, roll, balance and turn them-selves upside down, working every muscle in the body and loving every minute of it. All you have to do is give this natural move-ment a name – yoga – and encourage it. In India, children are taught yoga from the age of three, but most western ashrams don't recommend any type of formal yoga for children under the age of seven.

Younger children lack the concentration span of teens and

adults, of course, so if you plan to buy them a mat and introduce a more formal yoga practice, you are going to need to keep it short and child-friendly.

One way we do this is to change the strange sanskrit names of the asanas or postures. Sarvangasana, or the shoulder stand, for example, becomes the Candle. Bahhda Konasana becomes the Butterfly (which you can practise, too, to help stop your own hips from becoming stiff), and it looks just like its name. Vrikshasana becomes the Tree pose, and will help build strength in the lower back and legs and teach your child to balance. Ushtraasana, which is wonderful for strengthening the back muscles and stretching the throat, chest, stomach and thighs, becomes the Camel pose. You can see what some of these poses or postures look like on pages 151 and 152.

Here's a simple 25-minute yoga practice which I do with my five-year-old daughter and which is tailored for kids under ten. If 25 minutes sounds too long, drop a couple of the postures or spend less time on the breathing exercise. The one thing you mustn't drop is the relaxation at the end, which is when the real work gets done. Remember, always do your family yoga in a special, clean and tidy place. Light a candle and burn some incense to set the mood, but for younger kids do keep it short and sweet.

The practice

Om: Sit cross-legged and **chant** 'om' together three times. Explain that this is like prayer which helps us think about what's really important in life – being with the people we love, doing our best and looking after ourselves. (3 minutes.)

The Staff Pose (Dandasana) or Sitting Tall: You need strong back muscles to sit with your legs spread out in front of you, your hands flat on the mat by the sides of the hips and the spine straight. Start every session this way to build this strength. (2 minutes.)

The Butterfly: Now demonstrate how you can bring the soles of the feet together and let the knees fall out to the sides to make the shape of a butterfly. The idea is for the knees eventually to reach the floor. This gets harder as kids get older and the hips get stiffer. If the hips are very stiff, prop a pillow or cushion under each knee to give them the feeling of a soft landing. (2 minutes.)

The Camel and the Child: Start in a comfy high kneeling position and balance the feet on the tips of the toes. Look back towards the heels and, one at a time, take hold of each ankle with each hand. Then take hold of your right heel with your right hand, the left heel with your left. Keep the feet on the ground and lift the hips up and forwards. If you all feel OK in this position, let the head relax back towards the heels. This is the **Camel**. Hold this for a minute or so and then come out carefully by bringing the head up, the body back up straight and both arms back to the front at the same time. Counter the pose by kneeling forward with the forehead on the ground, the arms resting gently along-side the body. This is the pose of **the Child**. (3 minutes.)

The Candle: Now lie down and get ready for the shoulder stand. The important thing here is to show your child how to take the weight of their inverted body in their hands and to keep the back straight. Make sure there's lots of soft mat and carpet under the shoulders for padding. Tell older children the higher they place their hands, the greater the support for the back. See page 152. (3 minutes.)

The Tree: Come up into standing and feel what it's like to stand on just one leg. Think about how strong this leg has to become to take the whole body weight. See page 152 for the full pose. (2 minutes, holding the balance for one minute each side.)

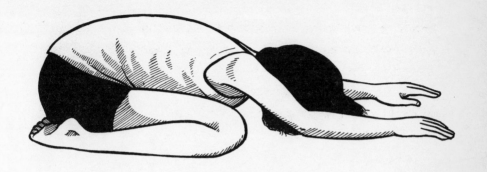

The Child

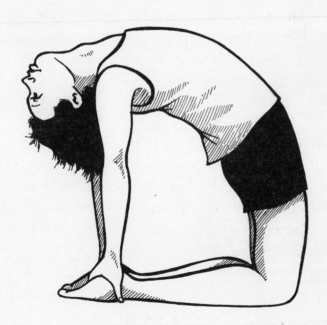

The Camel

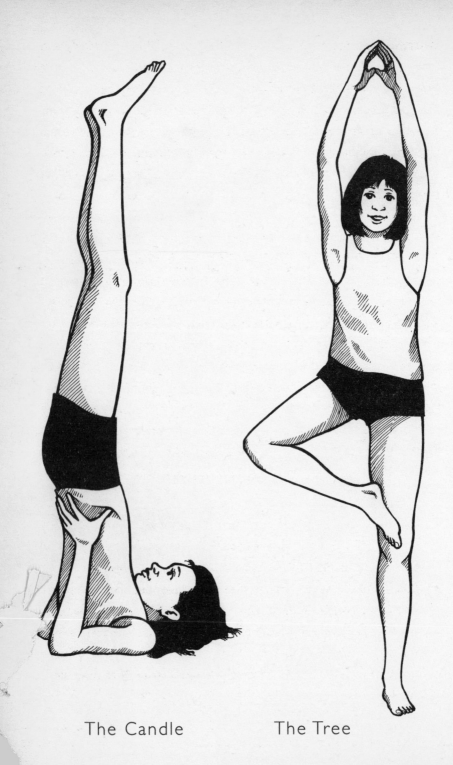

The Candle   The Tree

152   WHAT REALLY WORKS FOR KIDS

Breath: The breath is very important in yoga and just thinking about the breath will help your child relax. Ask them to lie down on the mat (eyes closed, legs slightly apart with the feet falling out to the sides), and then to imagine a big balloon in their tummy which fills up with air every time they breathe in, and which deflates again when they breathe out. Get them to really feel this balloon in their tummy and watch how their abdomen then rises and falls and how the breath deepens and slows down. (5 minutes.)

Relaxation: Always end with a peaceful relaxation. Still lying down, ask your child or children to forget their body and think about what is happening inside, in their head. Use this time to help build self-esteem or to tackle specific issues you know have been worrying them. Kids love visualization (which is like a bedtime story with your eyes closed) so tell them to imagine a big, strong, friendly tree either at the bottom of the garden or in the park and to imagine they can hang all their worries on this tree which will then take care of them. Get them to think about each worry they are handing over to the tree and explain that when they leave the tree those worries stay behind – gone for ever. You can help set the mood by playing peaceful music but don't play anything with words for them to latch on to and get distracted by. (5 minutes.)

*****

Five-star Tip

Want a good book? Try *The Complete Idiot's Guide to Yoga With Kids* (Alpha Books). The photos let the book down but the text and explanations are excellent. *Fly Like a Butterfly* by Skakta Kaur Khalsa has better pictures and some good meditations for relaxation. This is a Canadian book published by Rudra Press. You can get both of these from **amazon.co.uk** or from the **Nutri Centre Bookshop** on 020 7323 2382.

PART THREE

Food Talk

Introduction

Where do you think children today get most of the vitamin C their bodies need for healthy growth and development? If you were born in the 1950s or 1960s, the answer for your generation would have been simple: from fruit and vegetables, of course. Today, you need to think again. Because today kids don't get the vitamin C their bodies need from food at all. The majority of them get it from soft drinks. What this confirms is what any mum or dad could have told you without carrying out a clinical trial or a nationwide survey – that it would be easier to stop the tide than to get children to eat the healthy foods we (and they) know they should be eating but which don't stand a chance against the nutritionally dubious but tasty delights of junk and highly processed food.

What has been researched is that kids who are banned by parents from eating rubbish are more likely to eat junk behind their backs than those for whom it isn't banned. If you want to improve your child's diet, you are going to have to be just as sneaky and learn to outmanoeuvre them. This is exactly what Food Talk will show you how to do.

So, first of all, don't make the mistake of banning junk food. Simply limit it to a once- or twice-a-week treat. Second, get yourself a blender and introduce your kids to Smoothies. You can make these so tasty they won't even know they're drinking something healthy. You can sneak all kinds of ingredients, from immune-boosting herbs to calcium-rich tofu, into your mix and, guess what?, they'll never even know.

The key to getting some real live health-boosting nutrients down your kids is to make it no big deal. For instance, don't make them the delicious Cocoa-colada Smoothie on page 196, make it for yourself. But make sure you slurp it (with all the right appreciative noises) in front of them and count how long it is before they want one too. This section is the ultimate cheating parents' guide to getting it right without sweating the small stuff. They want chips? Fine, but read pages 163–4 before you decide what kind. Your toddler wants a snack? Great. Turn to page 165.

We all know we're supposed to be eating five healthy portions of fruit and veg each day (that's five combined, not five of each) and we all know most of us fail miserably. If we can't get that right, how can we expect our kids to? To make eating fruit and vegetables more fun, we've included a clever list of Rainbow Foods, where you can work out the health benefits by the colour of the food. Then invest in the Rainbow Food Activity Chart (see page 213) and learn how, by involving the whole family in a weekly Rainbow Food competition, you can all be winners in the healthy-eating stakes.

For those of you who like cooking (and for those who don't, why not give the kids the supervised run of the kitchen sometimes?), there are brand new Rainbow Recipes, including healthier versions of old favourites. Captain Hook's Hand of Cod should prove a talking point for all ages and the sugar-free

Raspberry Jelly Secrets are posh enough to serve at an adult dinner party.

Food Talk not only shows you how to cheat and sneak good food into your kids, it will remind you how much fun you can have while you're doing it. And you don't have to be a domestic goddess, a Delia or a Jamie to get the hang of it. In fact, if you follow our recipe for Simple Ten-Step Sushi – which the kids will love – you'll probably find it's not an inner child who's been hiding inside, it's a flamboyant family chef with a devoted following among . . . your own kids!

What do Kids Eat?

The short and not-so-sweet answer to this question is . . . rubbish. According to worried nutritionists, food diaries of teenagers, for example, show how it is not untypical for a seven-day diary covering twenty-one meals to include almost **no vegetables, fruits** or **water**. In Australia, researchers at the Flinders University School of Medicine looked at the diets of some 3,000 youngsters aged two to eighteen and concluded that not only do intakes of fruit and veg fall way below the recommended five portions per day; intakes have declined dramatically in the last decade. And the situation is no better here where, according to a survey carried out by the Cancer Research Campaign, hundreds of thousands of eleven- to sixteen-year-olds eat no fruit or vegetables at all most weeks.

Here is something else that will leave every parent who cares about their child's health in a state of shock. When scientists at the Human Nutrition Research Centre in Cambridge compared children's diets today with those of the relatively austere post-war 1950s, they found:

- In 1950, children got their iron from red meats. Today, they get it from fortified (and often high sugar) breakfast cereals.
- In 1950, children got their vitamin C from vegetables. Fifty years on, they get it from soft drinks.

With a diet that comprised more nutritious bread, more vegetables, less sugar, more fibre and fewer soft drinks, the nutritionists concluded the 1950s diet was more in line with current thinking about healthy eating than the food we are feeding children today. And this was their conclusion despite the fact the 1950s diet was higher in fat (presumably because back then kids ran around to burn off excess calories).

Even if today's children and their parents are trying to make healthy food choices, it can feel like an uphill struggle without a map. In recent months, foods as varied as baked beans and substitute butter spreads have been highlighted as being more of a health hazard than parents could ever have imagined. Even milk – that staple of childhood – has come under attack for sometimes being contaminated with a debilitating organism called *Mycobacterium avium paratuberculosis* (MAP), a strain of TB which has been linked with digestive problems in children, including Crohn's disease. And even if you reject this link as unproven, as a responsible parent you should be asking questions about traces of hormones in milk and what happens when these get into your child's body.

Sandwich spreads claiming to be healthier than butter have been found to contain harmful trans-fats, substances that form when polyunsaturated oils are cooked at high heat or hydrogenated, and which are as unhealthy (if not more so) as the saturated fats from meat and high-fat dairy foods. But perhaps the most alarming concern is that over the so-called gender-bending chemicals, linked to both cancer and damaged sexual development in kids, which have been identified in everyday foods ranging from canned beans to fish.

Teach your Kids to Cook

The best way to avoid a lot of the food hazards that have hit the headlines in recent months is to get back into the kitchen where you can teach yourself (if you were born after the 1960s) and the kids to cook. I'm not suggesting you chain yourself to the kitchen sink to become yet another domestic goddess, but cooking with and for the family really can be fun! Not only will it give you all real quality time together, you'll get a chance to experiment with all the fabulous, often exotic fresh produce now widely available in our supermarkets and you will know more about what you are actually eating. For families trying to cut back on additives (see page 34) and other unsavoury treats, this is the best way to know what's really in the food on your dinner plates.

Start with salads and sandwiches and progress to soups and the main meal. I believe there's no good reason why a child of ten cannot make the family meal and love doing it too. I always take my daughter food shopping with me. It should be fun and interesting and not some nightmare chore squashed in between the school run and the gym.

We Are What We Eat – Bioavailability

New research also shows how cooking vegetables makes the nutrients more bioavailable – bad news for those stalwart raw-fooders but excellent news for kids who mostly hate salads and anything that even looks healthy. Researchers at the vitamin and mineral laboratory of the Beltsville Human Nutrition Centre in America, for instance, have shown how the vitamin C in broccoli is more bioavailable once the vegetable has been cooked than when it is raw, and scientists at the Department of Foods and Nutrition at the Haryana Agricultural University in India who looked at protein intake from raw and cooked foods found that the digestibility, the biological value and the utilizable protein levels all improved after cooking. Other researchers working in East Africa have shown, too, how both blanching and cooking increase the concentration of cancer-preventing carotenoids in foods as diverse as peanuts and pumpkins.

Cooking does, of course, destroy some nutrients – especially vitamin C – but it also breaks down the cellulose structure of food to make the nutrients more available and the food more digestible. The best way to retain the vitamins and freshness of a vegetable is to steam it or, if you don't have a steamer, to cook it for a short time in only a little water over direct heat. This may be fine for adults, but for children who prefer a sweeter taste, you may need to compromise in the kitchen by cooking vegetables more slowly over a lower heat in order to make them more appetizing. If you avoid overcooking you can still preserve some 90 per cent of the nutrients and those you do lose, such as vitamin C, are easily replaced using herbs that are rich in that nutrient, e.g. parsley for vitamin C, as a garnish. In our house, we use simple and inexpensive steamers which sit over the saucepans and which enable us to preserve most of the micronutrients and taste of our vegetables.

*****

Five-star Tip

Re-use vegetable waters in soups, sauces and veggie juices to benefit from those nutrients that have leached out into the cooking pot.

Cooking also destroys parasites and amoebae which could otherwise enter the digestive system through raw food – an extra burden that the immature immune systems of growing children do not need.

The Scientist and the Potato Chip

Boiled and mashed potatoes have the highest and fastest digestibility according to Spanish researchers but of course the way most youngsters like their potatoes is straight from the chip pan. The task now ahead of scientists, like those at the Department of Food Biosciences at Reading University who are studying the uptake of fat by chipped potatoes, is to work out how to make the chip more healthy. What they have discovered is that during frying very little oil comes into contact with the chip and so very little oil is absorbed. It is when the chips come out of the pan that the problems start. And understanding how oil is absorbed by chips is, of course, the first step towards minimizing the problem and making a tasty low-fat version. Until we know more, the best way to reduce some of the fat uptake by chips is to quickly drain them straight from the pan onto kitchen paper before serving hot.

Here's the good news for parents whose chip-mad kids turn their noses up at all those so-called healthy foods (a term that in itself suggests that other foods are positively unhealthy):

- Brown rice may not, after all, have the edge over white.
- Not all fried foods are a heart attack waiting to happen.
- There is life – and ice cream – after a wheat or dairy intolerance!

When Portuguese researchers compared the nutritional value of brown rice with that of white they were surprised to discover that, although brown rice has a higher nutritional content, experimental data does not provide any evidence that a brown-rice diet is better than one based on white rice. The working theory is that brown rice may also contain antinutritional factors which have an adverse effect on the bioavailability of the nutrients in this cereal.

UK researchers setting out to find out whether all fried foods are bad for you examined how nutrients are lost and gained during the frying process, and concluded that this method of cooking has little or no detrimental impact on the nutritional status of the food. The amount of vitamin C in French fries, for instance, compared favourably with the amount in a raw potato. This paper also concluded that while some of the important antioxidant nutrients in food are lost during frying, this method of cooking has no impact on vitamin E – a fat-soluble nutrient which protects other nutrients, including vitamin C, from oxidation, and which can help protect children's lungs from the effects of pollution, prevent thick scar formation (inside the body and on the skin) and accelerate healing.

The Oxford Brookes University scientists concluded that fried foods are generally a good source of vitamin E and that, since they are highly palatable too, they have an important place in our diet. This, however, needs to be tempered by the knowledge that heating fats to high temperatures will also result in the formation of harmful trans-fats which can damage tissues. The solution? Try not to introduce fried foods to your children too early, if at all. And if they do develop a taste for them, serve them only occasionally.

Finally, life after food intolerances (see page 169). I have tracked down a delicious ice cream made from flaked oats and enriched with calcium. Called First Glace, it comes in vanilla, strawberry, chocolate and, for those who can't choose, vanilla-chocolate-fudge-swirl varieties and contains no additives or artificial ingredients. The oats make it a high-fibre pudding and it won't trigger the production of mucus and runny noses in sensitive kids. Visit **www.first-foods.com** to find stockists in your area.

Snack Attack

Researchers at the University of Carolina's Department of Nutrition studied the snacking habits of more than 20,000 youngsters aged between two and eighteen and then compared them with eating habits five and twenty years previously. They found that snacking has become more prevalent – that kids are getting more of their energy intake from snacks not meals – and warned that the snack is here to stay. The bad news for parents is that kids are snacking on high-energy sweets, prompting the researchers to call for a wider choice of healthier snackfoods. One way around this is to be prepared and make your own.

Get younger kids back into the healthy fruit snack habit by digging that old 1970s melon baller out from the back of the drawer and making melon or avocado mini-footballs. Melons are rich in vitamin C and carotenoids. Avocado is one of nature's own superfoods – the perfect ratio of fat, carbohydrate and protein and an excellent source of the omega-6 fatty acids that are involved in many body systems from maintaining healthy skin to regulating teen hormones.

You can even turn Kitchen Doctor and turn a snack attack to your advantage by choosing foods that can, say, boost the immune system to ward off bugs, bolster flagging concentration levels during exam time or lift energy levels when the going gets tough. For example, try these:

Bug-busting Snack – Monster Honey & Fig Bar

Honey – which was used for wound-healing before antibiotics – has such powerful antibacterial properties that it is now licensed for medical use in Australian hospitals. The most potent form is manuka honey, which is made by bees collecting their pollen from the tea tree plant and which is now widely on sale in health stores.

25g (1oz) soya spread

100g (3½oz) dried figs, chopped

25g (1oz) shelled pistachios

100g (3½oz) white flour

½ tsp baking powder

100g (3½oz) honey

1 tsp vanilla essence

2 eggs, beaten

25g (1oz) peanuts

What you do

1) Melt the soya spread and then mix with the other ingredients. Line a baking tray with greaseproof paper, pour the mixture in and spread evenly with a palette knife. Cook in an oven preheated to 180°C/350°F/Gas 4 for 20–25 minutes, until golden.

2) Leave to cool for 10 minutes, then cut into large breakfast bars. When completely cold, wrap each bar individually for school lunchboxes and snack attacks.

Brainbox Snack

Mash ½ a creamy ripe avocado (rich in omega-6 fatty acids) with ½ a smoked mackerel (rich in omega-3 fatty acids) to make a spread for a sandwich, rice cake or toast; a filling for jacket potatoes, or a home-made mini fishcake. The creaminess of the avocado cuts through the distinctive taste of the mackerel, making it more acceptable to the younger palate.

Erick's Energy Snack – Pea Bombs

These little green energy-bombs otherwise known as peas contain vitamin B1 (thiamine) which the body uses to convert the carbo-hydrates in food into energy; plus pantothenic acid, a member of the B-complex family, that helps convert other nutrients to energy. You might think you've no idea how to cook pulses or legumes but once you realize peas belong to this same family, there should be no stopping you. You can use this same recipe which is, in effect, a risotto (and which my French brother-in-law Erick devised for his children, Tiana and Mila), to disguise all manner of healthy veg!

90ml (3 fl oz) olive oil

1 large onion, finely chopped

2 garlic cloves, crushed

75g (2¾oz) carrots, peeled and grated

300g (10½oz) Italian arborio rice

900ml (1½ pints) vegetable stock, hot

140g (5oz) frozen peas or shelled, cooked garden peas

2 large tomatoes, skinned, deseeded and chopped

50g (1¾oz) fresh Parmesan cheese, grated

5 tbsp chopped fresh parsley

2 eggs, beaten

80g (3oz) polenta flour

What you do

1) Pour half the olive oil into a large saucepan and cook the onion and garlic until softened. Add the grated carrots and cook for another five minutes.

2) Add the uncooked arborio rice and cook for 2 minutes, stirring to coat every grain. Begin slowly to add the hot vegetable stock, a ladleful

at a time, stirring between each addition and allowing the stock to be absorbed.

3) After 10 minutes, add the peas and tomatoes. Season to taste and slowly add the rest of the vegetable stock, stirring continuously until the rice is cooked. It will look puffy and creamy. Now add the grated Parmesan cheese and chopped parsley. Leave to cool.

4) When the rice is cold, use your hands to make small bombs, no bigger than a medium-sized egg. Dip each one in the beaten egg and roll in polenta flour. Fry each energy bomb in the remaining olive oil until golden all over. Remove from the oil, drain, cool and store in an airtight container until the next snack break.

Take Five!

Here are my top ten tips for getting more healthy foods – snacks and meals – down the throats of junk-food-mad kids. Aim for five portions (combined, i.e. fruit or vegetable) a day but don't beat yourself up when you fall short. Remember, it is easier to incentivize younger kids (see page 196 for Rainbow Foods and details of the Rainbow Foods Activity Chart).

1 Throw out the Mighty White sugar-packed white bread (if you don't believe me, leave a small piece to soak under your tongue and see how sweet it tastes) and, instead of a limp sandwich, serve a wholemeal muffin turned into a mini pizza with home-made tomato topping (see page 215 for recipe), olives for the eyes and a slice of red pepper for the mouth.
2 Make your own hummus (see page 220) and stuff the bottom of a pocket-sized wholemeal pitta bread with alfalfa sprouts before

piling the hummus on. For teens, add a pinch of cayenne pepper for extra bite.

3 In winter, serve hot corn-on-the-cob dripping with melted almond butter from the health store. In summer, let the kids smear almond butter on slices of apple.

4 Julienne raw carrot into long thin strips to dip into runny eggs.

5 Make frozen fruit yoghurt pops to keep in the freezer. Just add puréed fruits to live plain yoghurt, find a good mould and freeze.

6 Purée fruits and veg to sneak onto the plate as sauces and side dishes. This is a brilliant way to get kids to eat some of the more unusual vegetables, such as sweet potatoes, fennel and celeriac.

7 Thicken sauces with vegetable purées instead of cream or milk.

8 Sneak vegetables into the noodles which kids love but save stir fries for an occasional treat since the high temperature will convert the fats in the oil into unhealthy trans-fats. Avoid this by steaming the vegetables first so they are almost cooked before hitting the wok. This means you don't have to turn up the heat.

9 Enhance the nutritional value of daily staples by adding fruits to everyday breakfast cereals, yoghurts and ice creams. In season, slice and serve them as a garnish and make purées to freeze.

10 Get a blender and become the Queen of Smoothies (see page 195).

Food Allergies and Food Intolerances

In the UK, government scientists have now stipulated that while the idea of food intolerances has become so fashionable that a third of the adult population believe themselves to be affected, only about 2 per cent of us genuinely do suffer from them. Poppycock. The human body was never designed for food technology or to keep eating the same highly processed wheat and dairy products, day in and day out. It is not that the body cannot digest wheat. It cannot digest what now passes for wheat in most commercial breads, pastries and high-tech foods. If you have a child plagued by a constantly runny nose, cut dairy products from their diet for a week and you will see just how quickly the body responds to what it gets to eat. (In this case, this is because dairy products, like their soy replacements, generate an overproduction of mucus in the body.)

Food intolerance is not, though, the same as a food allergy. If your child has the latter you will already know it. With an allergy, the body mistakenly identifies a food substance as a toxic invader. The immune system goes into overdrive and the body's own white blood cells end up doing more damage than the offending substance. Food intolerance is simply the inability of the body to properly digest a given food. What happens is that undigested particles of food enter the bloodstream through the gut wall and start to cause problems. The main culprits are always – without exception – wheat, dairy products and citrus fruits, and, for older children who may be drinking them, tea and coffee.

What causes a food intolerance in the first place is usually damage to the lining of the intestine. In perfect health, this acts like a filter, allowing nutrients through and keeping toxins and undigested food particles out of the bloodstream. It has small holes which do this job. If these enlarge – and this can be caused by, say, the prolonged use of antibiotics or by infections – they stop acting as a filter. This is a condition called leaky gut and, in many clinical trials, it has now been implicated in asthma, eczema and autism, following vaccination. Other signs of a food intolerance problem are irritable bowel syndrome, bloating and excessive tiredness.

Aloe vera* juice has a powerful healing action on the gut but

*Do not give aloe vera internally to kids under the age of twelve.

the flavour is not one most kids will relish. One of the best ways to disguise the taste is to hide the juice in a delicious fruit smoothie. (See page 196 for the Cocoa-colada which has such a rich flavour it will mask the taste of the aloe vera.) Aim to serve the equivalent of a quarter of a glass per day to kids over the age of twelve. For younger kids with digestive problems, use flaxseed (see page 104) or slippery elm in tincture form.

Who can test your child?

There are companies which test for food intolerances – although some of them charge up to £300, which is a bit steep. Some clinics use Vega or Mora Therapy machines and test for food intolerance as part of an initial assessment. Any qualified nutritionist can arrange for testing to be done. To find a practitioner in your area, call one of the following groups and ask for the names of those who specialize in child health:

- **The Institute of Optimum Nutrition (020 8877 9993).**
- **The British Association of Nutritional Therapists on 0870 6061284. (You will be charged £2 for a referral list.)**
- **The British Naturopathic Association on 01458 840072 holds a list of qualified naturopaths.**

Get to Grips with Exotic Grains

There are plenty of alternatives to wheat. The trouble is, even if we recognize them in the shop, lots of us just don't know what to do with them to make them tasty. Here are some tips to get you started.

Quinoa – more calcium than milk

A staple of the Inca diet and a cousin of the amaranth grain, quinoa has so many health-promoting properties that traditional South American cultures called it 'the mother grain'. It has the highest protein content of all grains – making it an excellent alternative for newly converted vegetarians and vegans who may still be craving protein. It also has more calcium than milk. A good source of blood-building iron, phosphorus for a healthy heart, kidneys and brain, antioxidant vitamin E and the antistress B vitamins, it has a higher fat content than other grains.

How to use it: Grind into a flour (I have an industrial strength juicer which also grinds grains) to use in baking breads and cakes or prepare in the same way as rice and serve in combination with other grains.

Amaranth – pop like popcorn!

In those African and South American cultures where this grain is still a staple, there is no malnutrition. Like quinoa, it contains more calcium than milk and it is also a good source of the co-nutrients magnesium and silicon which the body needs to make the best use of the calcium. It is also high in the amino acid lysine which can protect against a herpes infection, and which promotes strong bones and healthy skin.

How to use it: Pop like popcorn, toast for a nutty flavour or sprout on a tray on the windowsill to use in salads. Grind for baking or prepare and serve as a substitute for rice.

Barley – roast before cooking

Use whole not pearl barley since it contains more fibre, twice the amount of calcium, three times the proportion of iron and 25 per cent more protein. Whole barley is easily digested but is also a mild laxative. Unless you are suffering from constipation, remove this property by roasting before cooking. Roasted barley which is then ground into a powder makes a good substitute for coffee and sprouted barley is used in Chinese medicine to strengthen digestion and help treat candida infections (see Yeast Infections, page 387).

How to use it: Add to soups, casseroles or stews. Boil and serve as rice but be prepared for a chewier taste.

Cornmeal – add a twist of lime!

Available as polenta, which is the coarse version, or cornflour in its finer form, cornmeal is ground maize. It is traditionally cooked by Native Americans with lime to compensate for the fact it is low in niacin or vitamin B3. A deficiency in this nutrient can cause a fatal wasting disease called pellagra, but the lime works to increase the body's ability to absorb niacin. Blue corn is indigenous to South America and is a staple for the Hopi and Navajo people. It has 21 per cent more protein, 50 per cent more iron and twice the manganese and potassium of the yellow or white varieties.

How to use it: Use cornmeal flour for bread or muffins. Polenta can be cooked in boiling water a bit like porridge and then served as a grain, or allowed to set and then sliced and grilled or fried.

Millet – sshh, don't tell Goldilocks!

Rich in tissue-strengthening silicon and a good source of protein, millet has an alkalizing effect on the body and so can help treat conditions like bad breath by halting the growth of oral bacteria, which prefer a more acid environment. It is useful for settling the stomach if you have diarrhoea, but roast the grains before cooking.

How to use it: Start the day with millet porridge. To serve as a grain, cook in the same way as rice. The more water you add, the softer the grain will be. To vary the taste, toast in a little oil before cooking.

Old-fashioned oats – slow cookers

An obvious but often overlooked alternative to wheat, oats not only have a calming effect on the body, they also work to strengthen cardiac muscles and keep blood-cholesterol levels low. Oats are also one of the richest sources of silicon (see page 86), which supports the connective tissues in the body.

How to use them: Everyone knows how to make porridge but did you know the longer you slow-cook the oats, the more nourishing the final dish will be? You can also use them in soups, puddings, breads, crusts, toppings and desserts. See page 164 for details of the oat ice cream I have tracked down.

Alternatives to Dairy Products

What you are trying to avoid is casein – a protein in milk which many children over the age of two have difficulty digesting. Almond milk, almond butter, tahini, rice milk, goat or sheep products, soy (but be warned, soy promotes mucus-production in the body and so can be as congesting as high-protein meat and dairy products) and nut milks (as long as there is no underlying allergy) are all excellent and easy substitutes.

Whatever it Takes . . . So Cheat!

Smart parents will put a juicer on their birthday or Christmas list. Scientists at the Department of Family and Preventative Medicine at the University of California in San Diego have now proved what naturopaths have long argued – that the very best way to get nutrients into adults and kids is to juice fruits and vegetables. The researchers measured blood levels of important antioxidants such as lycopene from tomatoes and carotene from carrots in female breast-cancer patients and found levels of all these protective nutrients were higher among those who juiced their fruit and vegetables than those who ate them either raw or cooked.

If the family budget cannot stretch to a juicer, at least get a blender (mine cost just £12) so you can make nutrient-rich smoothies and shakes (see page 195).

The Ultimate Cheat!

KidGreenz is a brilliant cheat for parents who just can't get their kids to eat healthy greens. These chewy tablets contain broccoli, spinach, carrot juice, brown rice, alfalfa and even wheatgrass juice, making them a vegetarian mum's dream. The tropical flavour beats the taste of limp old spinach, making these a firm favourite in our household. Made by Nature's Plus, 60 chewable tablets cost £6.55. Mail-order from the **Nutri Centre** on 020 7436 0422 if not on sale in your local health store.

Synergy – FoodMates

Nutrients work together in the body and the clever family cook can easily learn which vitamins and minerals are the happiest bedfellows and how they work together in the body to enhance the action of each other. This is what nutritionists call synergy (see page 88 for supplements and synergy). And it works in two ways. First, certain nutrients enhance each other's action in the body. Secondly, you can serve FoodMates to make sure the body maintains its natural mild acidity and does not become overacidic, which can lead to health problems including headaches, sleeplessness and joint pains in adult life.

Nutrient synergy

Vitamin C, for example, is always more potent in the presence of substances called **bioflavonoids.** These give fruits and vegetables their glorious colours and, as well as their cancer-fighting properties – the bioflavonoid quercetin, for example, has been shown to inhibit the growth of cancer tumours – they all have an anti-inflammatory, antibacterial effect in the body where they work to promote healthy circulation, stimulate bile production for the breakdown of fats in food and lower blood-cholesterol levels.

Foods that are rich in bioflavonoids include apples, beetroot, blackberries, blackcurrants, cabbage, carrots, cauliflower, cherries, dandelions, lemons, lentils, lettuce, oranges, parsley, plums, peas, potatoes, rhubarb, rose hips, spinach, tomatoes, walnuts and watercress. And all these have even more potency when eaten with vitamin C (and vice versa).

Synergistic partners are rarely monogamous. Quercetin, for example, is synergistic with vitamin C but also with an anti-inflammatory enzyme called bromelain which is found in fresh pineapple (see page 205). Vitamin C-rich citrus fruits such as lemon and lime also work well with iron-rich green vegetables since vitamin C can boost iron absorption by up to 30 per cent – a synergistic relationship that is even more important for children who, ideally, need to get their iron supplies from food not supplements, since any excess iron will be stored in the liver.

Acid/Alkaline Synergy

FoodMates can also work together in the body to maintain the all-important acid/alkaline balance which, when out of kilter, can adversely affect both the skin and the digestive tract and which should work to fight off those external infections which have been implicated in skin problems such as acne and eczema. Acidity and alkalinity are measured according to the pH (which stands for potential of hydrogen) scale. Water, which has a pH of 7.0, is neutral – neither acid nor alkaline. A pH below 7.0 is acidic, and anything with a pH higher than 7.0 is alkaline. The human body is naturally mildly acidic in order to resist infection – its ideal pH is between 6.0 and 6.8. Acidosis is the medical term for an imbalance where the body chemistry has become over-acidic. As well as skin and digestive disorders, symptoms of this imbalance can include insomnia, headache and joint pains.

Serving acid foods with alkaline ones can help maintain the correct and healthy pH balance. The alkaline properties of a mango, for instance, will counter the high acidity of strawberries and so can help prevent any adverse reaction if you eat them both together. Nutmeg and mushrooms make unusual but effective FoodMates since nutmeg is a natural antibacterial and will counter the effects of any infection lurking in the bacteria-prone fungus. Serve alkaline almonds or other nuts with spicy foods to neutralize the acidity of the dish, and serve pizza with garlic bread which contains sulphur to deactivate the yeast action of the pizza's dough base.

Sugar, fish, chicken, noodles and eggs – food staples for many children – are all acid-forming foods. Fresh vegetables, coconut, maple syrup, honey, raisins and soy products are all alkaline-forming foods. So noodles served with stir-fried broccoli, carrots and a splash of soy sauce is the perfect balance.

Complete Proteins

For parents of vegetarian children and those avoiding certain foods because of an intolerance (see page 169), the idea of FoodMates takes on even more significance. Here you can learn how to combine foods to make what are called complete proteins. Most of us eat twice as much protein as we actually need, so the key for good health is to eat the right type of healthier proteins (e.g. from beans not high-fat animal meats) in the right proportions. Proteins are made up of smaller units called **amino acids**. There are twenty-two of these, fourteen of which the body can make. The other eight, called the essential amino acids, must come from diet. Animal and dairy products provide all eight but plant foods do not, which is where clever food combining, especially for vegetarian kids, takes centre stage.

Cashew butter on wholegrain bread, for example, will provide all eight essential amino acids, so will wholewheat pasta with sautéed pine nuts, vegetables and Parmesan cheese. Meatless chilli with brown rice will work and so will tortilla with beans – that staple of the Mexican diet. Remember the cheese and pineapple sticks that your parents served at cocktail parties in the 1970s? High-fat proteins such as cheese, yoghurt and nuts* make good FoodMates with acid fruits such as pineapple, kiwi, strawberries and oranges.

*Do not use nuts if there is any underlying allergy.

At-a-Glance FoodMates

- **Apple & Pumpkin Seeds**
- **Pizza & Garlic Bread**
- **Cheese & Pineapple**
- **Chocolate & Pears**
- **Cow's Milk & Nutmeg**
- **Curry & Almonds**
- **Peanuts & Turmeric**
- **Oranges & Sunflower Seeds**
- **Strawberries & Mango**
- **Cashew Butter & Wholegrain Bread**
- **Meatless Chilli & Brown Rice**
- **Tortilla & Beans**
- **Yoghurt & Kiwi Fruit**

Food Rage
. . . or why you need to know about the Glycaemic Index (GI)

The Glycaemic Index may sound like a boring old medical term but it is much more relevant to family life than you think. When Dad starts ranting in a traffic jam or little Johnny starts stabbing the table with his straw in McDonald's, it's not bad manners or a filthy temper to blame but a slump in blood sugar levels and a Food Rage.

This condition – the symptoms of which include frayed nerves, hunger pangs, fatigue, a short temper and feelings of pent-up aggression – is called hypoglycaemia, or low blood sugar, if it persists. Thankfully, for most of us, eating will soon banish these symptoms by sending blood sugar levels back to normal. The trouble is that if you eat or give the kids foods that release sugar very quickly, you may be setting up a cycle of blood sugar highs and lows which will carry on affecting behaviour and mood throughout the day.

This is where the Glycaemic Index (GI) comes in. This is a system of ranking foods according to how quickly or slowly they affect blood sugar levels. Scientists, who started by giving a ranking of 100 for white bread, have now assessed some 600 different foods according to the rate of their impact on blood sugar and compared them with this staple. All the ranked foods are carbohydrates since these are the main source of glucose (blood sugar) in the body.

Once you've mastered the GI theory – which is simply to eat foods which rank at 50 or below – you can introduce the GI way of eating at home and, hopefully, bid goodbye to food rages, road rages, temper tantrums, squabbling and other signs of low blood sugar levels.

It's also fascinating to note that with this system, so-called health foods which taste like old cardboard may not be as good for you as you think. Take rice cakes, that staple of the health guru cupboard. Rice has a high GI to give an instant energy hit and so according to the index a rice cake (ranking 77) is less healthy than a slice of sponge cake (ranking 47). French fries are 'healthier' than brown rice. Skimmed milk is ranked higher than full-fat milk. And, believe it or not, even crisps at 54 work out healthier than high-sugar dates which rank a massive 99.

According to GI eaters, it is also better to eat five smaller meals, at regular intervals and made up of foods ranked lower than 50, than to eat three big meals a day. This is good news for grazers and snackers as long as the foods are from the lower end of the GI scale.

At-a-Glance Guide to the GI of Kids' Foods

White bread: 100

Rice Krispies: 82

Cooked carrots: 85

Baked potato: 85

White rice: 81

Brown rice: 76

French fries: 75

Crumpets: 69

Boiled potatoes: 63

Ice cream: 61

Pitta bread: 57

Rich tea biscuits: 55

Macaroni: 49

Baked beans: 48

Green peas: 48

Mixed grain breads: 46

Spaghetti: 41

Apples: 38

Fish fingers: 38

Tomato soup: 38

Low-fat yoghurt: 33

Skimmed milk: 32

Sausages: 28

Full-fat milk: 27

Kidney beans: 27

- To learn more about GI eating, read *The Glucose Revolution* by Dr Anthony Leeds, Professor Jennie Miller et al. Published by Hodder & Stoughton, it costs £10 and includes recipes and simple GI charts. Remember, though, that low-ranking GI foods can be high in unhealthy saturated fats (e.g. sausages) and additives (e.g. baked beans, fish fingers) so, again, balance, variation and moderation are key.

The HealthClub Bouncers

In children, you are building long-term health and immunity against disease and, to do this, your best food allies are the **antioxidant nutrients**. These are the **vitamins A, C and E** (**ACE**), plus the new kid on the block **selenium**. (New because it has only just been given an adult RNI.)

Lots of people bandy the term 'antioxidant' around but have little idea what it means. An antioxidant is any substance that protects the body from free radicals – the extra oxygen molecules that are produced naturally when our cells produce energy, and less naturally when we are exposed to harmful pollutants and toxins in the environment and in food. One easy way to get the idea is to liken these free radicals to groups of marauding drunks trying to barge their way into Stringfellows, and to think of the antioxidants as the burly bouncers keeping them out.

Other potent antioxidants are the **betacarotenes** which the body uses to make vitamin A and other **carotenoids** such as lycopene, which gives tomatoes their red colour, and lutein, an anti-cancer agent found in spinach. The **bioflavonoids** which give fruits and vegetables their fabulous colours were dismissed until recently as being little more than natural food dyes. Now we know these too have powerful antioxidant and often anti-inflammatory properties. They include substances such as **quercetin** in red onions, and rutin, which is found in citrus fruits and is excellent for keeping blood vessels healthy.

Left unchecked, the unstable free radicals can harm healthy tissues but antioxidants prevent this by binding with them before they can do any serious damage. We measure antioxidants in units known as Oxygen Radical Absorbance Capacity (ORAC), which means you can then not only identify those foods with good antioxidant action but single out those that perform this function best in the body. Among the antioxidant fruits, the top-scoring ORACs per 100g (3½oz) serving are not always the most obvious. They are:

prunes (5770)
raisins (2830)
blueberries (2400)
blackberries (2036)
strawberries (1540)
raspberries (1220)

With vegetables, the top-scorers are:

kale (1770)
spinach (1260)
Brussels sprouts (980)
alfalfa sprouts (930)
broccoli (890)
beetroot (840)

Cooking with Phytopharmaceuticals
(that's herbs again)

A herb is any plant that has a medicinal action in the body, and the more you research this area, the more you realize that every plant has some action – good or bad. Herbal medicine has become so popular in Britain that we now buy more herbal remedies than any other country. And an excellent place to start using herbs is in the family kitchen. You won't be using dosages large enough to cause any harmful side effects and as well as improving the flavour of your foods, you will be incorporating new and often unimagined health benefits when you add a pinch of chopped parsley or a sprig of roughly cut sage.

Parsley, Sage, Rosemary and . . . Wolfberry

In my kitchen, everyday herbs such as parsley and thyme have to fight for space with the rather more exotic-sounding Indian herbs such as asafoetida, which we use in place of garlic, and the Chinese staples astragalus and wolfberry. Recent scare stories about Chinese herbs have been wildly exaggerated and the only thing you need to do is to make sure the herbs you are buying and using in both cooking and herbal teas are not suitcase imports but come from a reputable supplier.

Don't let strange and unfamiliar names frighten you off using herbs you have not heard of before. Some of the health benefits are astounding. Asafoetida, for instance, is used in Ayurvedic medicine (see page 133) to eliminate stagnant waste from the intestinal tract and is especially good at clearing out the toxins and impacted waste that can be the result of a heavy meat or junk food diet. Similar to garlic but stronger, cook it with lentils and beans to make them more digestible and to reduce gas. It can be used to help relieve flatulence, abdominal pains and digestive disorders, and will kick-start peristalsis to prevent constipation. In Ayurvedic medicine, asafoetida is said to ignite and strengthen Agni – the digestive fire that keeps the body and the emotions healthy.

In Traditional Chinese Medicine (TCM – see page 130), food therapy is an important treatment tool and many of the herbs that offer the best health benefits have wonderful names like the red wolfberry (lychee berries), which always makes me think of Little Red Riding Hood, and the lotus seed, which is used to 'nourish the heart and calm the spirit'. The idea is that you can use food and herbs to correct any imbalance betwen the yin and yang opposites – hot and cold; sweet and salty; damp and dry; slow and fast – that may be causing specific health conditions or that may just be leaving you or the kids feeling under par.

TCM categorizes and then uses herbs according to whether, for example, they have a heating or cooling effect in the body, whether they are sweet or sour, whether they will mobilize the life force or chi in the blood and whether they can help rid the body of damp, which is a common problem for families living in the UK climate. TCM also considers the effects each herb will have on the body's subtle energies and spiritual nature.

I was first introduced to cooking with Chinese herbs by a London-based GP, Dr Shamim Dyer, who now runs a series of short residential food therapy courses* throughout the year in the UK. If you can sign up for one, then do, and watch your confidence in using unusual herbs in your cooking grow overnight. Until then, here's a taster of the health benefits of some of the more exotic herbs you can introduce at home. You can even mix two or three together. We often tie liquorice, a dozen or so wolf-berries and a slice or two of astragalus in a small square of muslin to drop into the casserole dish when we are slow-cooking a winter stew, but you can use these herbs in porridges and sauces too. The packets will give an idea of how much to use but, as with the western herbs we use, we favour the chuck-it-in-and-see method.

*For details of Dr Shamim Dyer's food therapy courses, call her clinic on 020 7580 7537. You can buy all these herbs from Chinese supermarkets or mail-order them in prepared packs for cooking from Dr Dyer on the same number. The Register of Chinese Herbal Medicine is on 0700 790332.

The exotic herbs

Astragalus Root: Has a sweet and slightly warming action which is used in TCM to help correct what practitioners call a spleen deficiency. (The spleen makes, stores and destroys red blood cells.) It can also help **relieve fatigue** and **bolster a poor appetite**.

Chrysanthemum Flower: Sweet and slightly cold, this herb works on the liver and the lungs and helps clear heat-related disorders such as **headaches** and **fevers**.

Lotus Seeds: These look like little off-white wooden beads that the kids might string together to make a necklace. Said to nourish the heart and calm the spirit, they can also help **prevent insomnia** and **soothe irritability**. They work on the kidney and heart energies.

Liquorice Root: Nothing like the long chewy black strings we used to buy from the sweetshop, when you buy this herb you get what looks like unappetizing slices of tree bark. Don't be put off. A fantastic immune-booster and wonderful for relieving **sore throats**, **respiratory problems** and **fatigue**, liquorice also works to help other herbs 'enter' into the energy channels so that they too will hit the spot.

Wolfberry: Sweet and said to tonify the liver and kidneys, these deep-red berries will also look great on the spice shelf. They can help **relieve mild stomach ache and lower back grumbles,** especially during menstruation when they also help to correct any blood deficiency.

Poria: Looks like dried-out old chalk – in fact, it is a mushroom – and comes in the pack in unappealing-looking flattened lumps but said to be brilliant for clearing the mind to **support the memory**, so an excellent herb to sneak into a supper dish during exam-time. Also works to promote **healthy digestion** and **keep the kids calm**.

Homegrown herbs and spices

Of course, you are unlikely to be growing exotic herbs in your own garden and even less likely to find them on sale in your own local supermarket. Everyday western herbs that you can grow – in pots on the windowsill or in your own herb garden – can also enhance not only the taste of your cooking but your family's health; especially when you know what medicinal properties they have and can take a more scientific overview.

Parsley: How boring is this herb? Not at all in fact. There are lots of different varieties – flat-leafed or curly – and they are all rich in protein, which is important for **building strong bones and muscles**, and in vitamins A, B complex, C and K (see Vitamins Guide, page 66). Parsley also has **mild antibacterial properties** and promotes **healthy digestion**.

Sage: Like strawberries, sage contains ellagic acid which can help **prevent damage to the cells' genetic material, DNA.** It has antimicrobial and antispasmodic action and was traditionally used to treat the **night sweats** in TB patients. Again, far from being a dull old herb, sage has such potent healing properties that it is now being investigated by phytopharmaceutical companies for the role it could play in preventing and treating Alzheimer's disease in adults by restoring the impaired vascular supply to the brain. It also works to **enhance memory**.

Rosemary: Not just a garnish for lamb but a powerful antioxidant which will help protect the body from damage by free radical molecules, rosemary is also a **good antidote to stress**.

Thyme: An excellent **aid to digestion**, thyme can help dislodge the mucus coating of the intestinal tract which would otherwise cause problems in the long term. It also has **antiseptic properties** and so is often used in more natural toothpastes.

Even a pinch of **kitchen cupboard spice**, such as cinnamon or all-spice, can claim significant health benefits. Spices contain natural chemicals called isothiocyanates which block carcinogens and suppress multiplication of any cells which may have taken those first steps towards becoming cancerous.

Substitute Meals

This is for children who say no to three square meals a day and mean it! With teenage eating disorders on the increase among boys as well as girls, food is a tricky issue in many households. One of the best ways to get healthy nutrients into your kids – especially faddy eaters and stroppy burger-mad teens – is to buy a blender and start making smoothies, which can easily be made nutritious and filling enough to substitute for meals. Here are the storecupboard staples you will need to make the best-tasting and most nutritious smoothies in the neighbourhood.

For flavouring

Organic maple syrup, coconut milk, organic cocoa powder, manuka honey, homemade organic fruit coulis and syrups. To make a coulis, simmer fresh fruit with an equal part of water, and honey to taste, until thickened. Strain, cool and use for natural flavouring.

For health kicks

Acidophilus powder: A probiotic designed to rebuild levels of the good bacteria that aid digestion. Can help boost immunity and is important to take after illness and prescription drugs, especially antibiotics (see page 95).

Flaxseed (linseed) oil or seeds: Not the kind you use for oiling cricket bats but the one on sale in health stores. Use to promote and maintain healthy digestion.

Aloe vera juice: Odd but not unpleasant-tasting rapid gut healer which can help kick-start sluggish bowels and keep digestion healthy. Again, on sale in health stores. Check the label and look for products with a high mucopolysaccharide content. If in doubt, mail-order your supplies from **Nature's Choice** on 020 8944 5584, which stocks the good quality Forever Young range. A litre, which should last three months, costs £14.95. Once opened, store it in the fridge.

- **Do NOT give aloe vera juice internally to children under twelve. You need only use these herbs until the digestive disorder has cleared. Flaxseed can help maintain healthy digestion. Give as directed on the label. For maintenance only, give half the age-appropriate dosage.**

Nuts and seeds: Almonds, cashews, sunflower, pumpkin and sesame seeds. All high in protein and rich in brain-boosting essential fatty acids. Will add a nutty taste and texture to smoothies. Cheat with **almond butter** from the health store.

- **Soaking nuts before blending activates the enzymes and makes them easier to digest.**

Dates: Packed with natural sugar for a quick energy hit, dates are the top-rated smoothie sweetener in our household. A mild laxative, they are a good source of the stress-busting B vitamins, plus calcium and magnesium.

Raisins: Gives the kids something to chew on and high in heart-protecting potassium.

Brewer's yeast: Rich in the B vitamins which support the nervous system, this energy-booster helps the body metabolize sugar and is useful in helping control eczema and promoting good sleep patterns.

Lecithin: Helps flush harmful fats from the body and may play a role in keeping the brain healthy. Widely available from health stores.

Wheatgrass: A superfood, no less. Tastes vile on its own – my little girl always says, 'Mummy, why are you eating grass?' – but that grassy flavour can be disguised with the addition of fresh mint to juiced wheatgrass, lemons and green apples.

Vitamin C and any other vitamin pill or herbal remedy: Smoothies are a great way to disguise the taste of herbs and nutritional supplements you may be using to tackle specific conditions. For instance, add vitamin C and echinacea tincture to beat a cold. Add a B-complex supplement and acidophilus in times of stress. In other words, make your own kitchen medicines.

The incredible bulking agents

Rice: The most easily digested of all the grains and the one least likely to trigger an allergic reaction. Technically brown rice is healthier because it has not been stripped of nutrients but researchers now believe it may also contain some antinutritional factor that closes the health gap with white rice (see page 163). We use both in smoothies.

Tofu: We use this ingredient more than any other in our smoothies. A complete protein, when blended it lends its creamy texture to these substitute meals. However, it creates more mucus in the body so switch to another agent for kids suffering from runny noses, hay fever and colds.

Millet: High in protein and carbohydrates, millet has a mild flavour and is also a rich source of silica which gives the lungs their elasticity, helps skin disorders, protects children's vulnerable ear, nose and throat passages, and boosts the absorption of other minerals.

Oat bran: High in fibre; naturopaths prescribe oat remedies for their calming action in the body. Oats can help lift depression and will also keep cholesterol levels low so you can use them to counter the more harmful effects of a high-fat meal later in the day.

Grape Nuts cereal: This toasted barley has both antioxidant and antiviral properties and so this is an excellent bulking agent if you are making an immune-boosting smoothie to ward off coughs and colds.

Fruits and Vegetables in Season

Eating with the seasons is not only one way to try to avoid some of the more hazardous food-processing techniques designed to extend shelf life, it also means your children will benefit from the nutrients in the most fresh foods. The only advantage with eating foods more than a day or two old is that older vegetables contain more insoluble fibre and so will provide more of what we used to call roughage. Try to eat produce that is in season by checking against this handy list supplied by the **Organic Delivery Company** (020 7739 8181). It is a list for pragmatic people, not purists. Sometimes an imported peach is better than no peach at all.

January: Apples, avocados, bananas, dates, grapefruit, black grapes, lemons, mangoes, oranges, pears, rhubarb, aubergine, raw beetroot, broccoli, carrots, cauliflower, green and white cabbages, celeriac, courgettes, fennel, ginger, leeks, mangetout

February: Apples, avocados, bananas, dates, white grapes, black grapes, lemons, mangoes, oranges, pears, aubergine, raw beetroot, broccoli, carrots, cauliflower, green and white cabbages, celeriac, courgettes, fennel, garlic, ginger, leeks, mangetout, sugarsnap peas

March: Apples, avocados, bananas, grapefruit, dates, white grapes, kiwi, lemons, mangoes, oranges, pears, aubergine, raw beetroot, broccoli, carrots, cauliflower, green and white cabbages, cherry tomatoes, celeriac, courgettes, fennel, garlic, ginger, leeks, mangetout, sugarsnap peas

April: Apples, avocados, bananas, grapefruit, dates, white grapes, kiwi, lemons, mangoes, oranges, pears, pineapple, aubergine, raw beetroot, broccoli, carrots, cauliflower, green and white cabbages, cherry tomatoes, celeriac, courgettes, fennel, garlic, ginger, leeks, mangetout, sugarsnap peas, spinach

May: Apples, avocados, bananas, grapefruit, dates, white grapes, kiwi, lemons, mangoes, oranges, pears, peaches, pineapple, papaya, aubergine, raw beetroot, broccoli, carrots, cauliflower, green and white cabbages, cherry tomatoes, tomatoes, celeriac, courgettes, fennel, garlic, ginger, leeks, mangetout, sugarsnap peas, spinach, celery, watercress

June: Apples, avocados, apricots, bananas, grapefruit, dates, white grapes, kiwi, lemons, mangoes, oranges, pears, peaches, pineapple, papaya, melon, limes, nectarines, plums, cherries, figs, raspberries, strawberries, aubergine, raw beetroot, broccoli, carrots, cauliflower, green and white cabbages, cherry tomatoes, tomatoes, celeriac, courgettes, fennel, garlic, ginger, leeks, mangetout, sugarsnap peas, spinach, celery, watercress

July: Apples, avocados, apricots, bananas, blueberries, watermelons, grapefruit, dates, peaches, white grapes, kiwi, lemons, raspberries, strawberries, mangoes, oranges, pears, peaches, pineapple, papaya, melon, limes, nectarines, plums, cherries, figs, aubergine, raw beetroot, broccoli, carrots, cauliflower, green and white cabbages, cherry tomatoes, tomatoes, celeriac, courgettes, fennel, garlic, ginger, leeks, mangetout, sugarsnap peas, spinach, celery, watercress

August: Apples, avocados, apricots, bananas, blueberries, watermelons, dates, peaches, kiwi, lemons, raspberries, strawberries, mangoes, oranges, pears, pineapple, papaya, melon, limes, nectarines, plums, cherries, figs, aubergine, raw beetroot, broccoli, carrots, cauliflower, green and white cabbages, cherry tomatoes, tomatoes, celeriac, courgettes, fennel, garlic, ginger, leeks, mangetout, sugarsnap peas, spinach, celery, watercress

September: Apples, avocados, apricots, bananas, blueberries, water-melons, grapefruit, grapes, dates, peaches, kiwi, lemons, raspberries, strawberries, oranges, pears, pineapple, papaya, melon, limes, plums, figs, aubergine, raw beetroot, broccoli, carrots, cauliflower, green and white cabbages, cherry tomatoes, tomatoes, celeriac, courgettes, fennel, garlic, ginger, leeks, mangetout, sugarsnap peas, spinach, celery, watercress, greens

October: Apples, avocados, bananas, blueberries, grapefruit, grapes, dates, kiwi, lemons, oranges, pears, pineapple, limes, plums, persimmons, aubergine, raw beetroot, broccoli, carrots, cauliflower, green and white cabbages, cherry tomatoes, tomatoes, celeriac, courgettes, fennel, garlic, ginger, leeks, mangetout, sugarsnap peas, spinach, celery, watercress, greens

November: Cranberries, apples, bananas, blueberries, grapefruit, grapes, dates, kiwi, lemons, oranges, pears, pineapple, limes, plums, figs, persimmons, rhubarb, aubergine, raw beetroot, broccoli, carrots, cauliflower, green and white cabbages, cherry tomatoes, tomatoes, celeriac, courgettes, fennel, garlic, ginger, leeks, mangetout, sugarsnap peas, spinach, celery, watercress, greens

December: Cranberries, apples, avocados, tangerines, mandarins, bananas, blueberries, grapefruit, grapes, dates, kiwi, lemons, oranges, pears, pineapple, limes, plums, figs, persimmons, rhubarb, aubergine, raw beetroot, broccoli, carrots, cauliflower, green and white cabbages, cherry tomatoes, tomatoes, celeriac, courgettes, fennel, garlic, ginger, leeks, mangetout, sugarsnap peas, spinach, celery, watercress, greens

Sticky Syrups and Slurps

Slowly simmer 100g/3½oz sugar with 120ml/4fl oz water until dissolved. Add 200g/7oz prepared fresh fruit, simmer for 15 minutes, strain, cool and store in the fridge. Dilute your syrup with filtered water to make a refreshing cold drink, or in milk to make a slurp. For a treat, blend with ice cream. Remember, the sugar content will be high, and although you'll know there's no aspartame or other nasty additives in the drink, you should still save it for an occasional treat.

Strawberry Slurp: Keep winter colds and flu away with an antiviral strawberry drink.

the kitchen and works like a star chart for good behaviour but with Power Animal stickers instead of stars (see page 213). The idea is for each family member to aim for at least five portions of fruit and vegetables (combined) from the following rainbow foods each day. Charting the health benefits of different foods by their colour is not only fun for kids, it makes it easier for mums and dads to remember which nutrients each food provides.

Red Foods

Tomatoes: It's not often that processed foods get a look in on the health pages but when it comes to tomatoes, cooked is even better than raw. The active ingredient is lycopene which gives tomatoes their red colour. This is a powerful antioxidant which can protect against disease but which is easier to absorb if the tomatoes have been processed. This is good news for toddlers and teens since it means both tomato ketchup and pizza sauce are more powerful antioxidants than the uncooked tomato in a salad. Said to cleanse the liver and purify the blood, tomatoes are also rich in vitamin C, which keeps the immune system strong. Tomato juice is acidic and so can help the body break down meat fibres during digestion. If you can get them, tomatoes which have been left to ripen on the vine are best.

Red peppers: If you think oranges are the best source of vitamin C, think again. Like tomatoes, red peppers contain lycopene, but one pepper also provides over 100 per cent of the RNI for vitamin C. In fact, red peppers provide all the antioxidants that are crucial for building health – vitamins A, C, E and selenium. The latter is especially important for males. In one trial, for example, adult men taking the equivalent of 159mcg of selenium a day had three times less risk of developing prostate problems than those not taking supplementation. The average intake of selenium for British males is just 86mcg per day.

Red kidney beans: A good source of iron, kidney beans are also packed with fibre – a half cup (100g or 3½oz) serving will provide more than 7g of fibre. They are also rich in potassium, which supports the heart, muscles and blood and which has been shown to be useful in the fight against eczema (see page 329). In Chinese medicine, kidney beans are used to nurture the kidneys. Team with rice in a vegetarian chilli dish to provide a complete protein meal for kids. To improve the flavour and digestibility of all beans, cook with a strip of kombu or kelp seaweed in the bottom of the pot.

Red onions: Long before we had over-the-counter cold remedies, herbalists would make a syrup of onions to treat colds and nasal congestion. And it worked. We now know that all onions are rich in a superstar bioflavonoid called quercetin which blocks the release of histamines – the proteins which cause all the symptoms of an allergic reaction, including runny noses, watery eyes and congestion. It also has strong anticancer properties. According to researchers at the Beijing Institute for Cancer Research, adults who ate a lot of quercetin-rich onions reduced their risk of cancer twenty-fold. Cooking does not destroy quercetin. Onions are also a good source of sulphur and can act in the body as natural antibiotics, helping to retard the growth of yeasts such as candida and fungi such as the organism responsible for athlete's foot.

Strawberries: Rich in vitamin C and fibre but also a fantastic source of ellagic acid – a powerful phytochemical which can block the action of carcinogens from food and the environment. As well as protecting the body from pollution and the ravages of stress, strawberries can help repair DNA damage in the cell. They contain pectin fibre and, gram for gram, are an even better source of fibre than wholegrain breads. Strawberries also act as antiviral agents and can help suppress the herpes virus which can cause cold sores (see page 311). They also provide silicon, which helps strengthen the connective tissue that connects bones to joints and the collagen that gives young skin its elasticity. Make a strawberry herbal tea or warm syrup to soothe sore throats but always sniff before you buy since if the berries have no smell, there will be no taste either, and watch out for imported, irradiated fruits.

Raspberries: High on flavour and low in calories, raspberries are also high in calcium and fibre. Like all red-skinned fruits, they act as natural antibiotics in the body where they can help alleviate diarrhoea and support the liver. A high vitamin C content provides an extra boost for the immune system. Make a cooling summer drink by adding ice cubes to tepid raspberry tea and serve fresh raspberries to a teen who is craving something sweet but trying not to gain weight.

Rhubarb: Everyone knows you get calcium from milk and yoghurt, but rhubarb is a superb source too. Just one cupful (200g/7oz) will give you a third of the recommended daily dose. It also contains manganese, which helps activate the enzymes the body needs to properly use vitamin C and biotin. This nutrient is important for kids since it is crucial for normal bone structure and for the proper digestion and utilization of food.

Watermelons: From the same family as pumpkins and cucumbers, all melons are natural diuretics and so will help prevent water retention in premenstrual daughters. Another excellent low-calorie food, it is better to eat watermelon before a meal or as a snack on its own since it is digested very quickly in the gut. What this means is that eating it with other food will slow this process down, leading to fermentation in the digestive tract. High in vitamin C and betacarotenes, a generous slice of watermelon will provide a good proportion of the RNI of both these nutrients. Watermelons are also high in potassium, which plays a role in the developing nervous system as well as supporting the heart, muscles, kidneys and circulatory systems. Potassium also helps clear the brain, making watermelon a wonderful snack for teens revising for summer exams.

Orange Foods

Carrots: A single carrot contains enough betacarotene – the anti-oxidant substance which protects against cellular damage and which the body converts to vitamin A – for one whole day. Vitamin A plays a key role in maintaining the health of the body's inner and outer membrane surfaces and so is useful in preventing respiratory and skin complaints. Carrots are rich in cellulose – a form of fibre which helps remove cancer-causing toxins from the colon wall. Sweet and nutritious for children, purée cooked carrots for toddlers and weaning infants, especially those in the throes of diarrhoea. After an attack, carrot soup can also help prevent dehydration. Carrots help stimulate appetite so tempt more faddy teens with a slice of homemade carrot cake. Carrots slow the progress of cancer in already damaged cells and so count as one of the Rainbow vegetable superstars. If juicing, one pound (almost half a kilogram) of carrots will produce one glass of carrot juice, which you then dilute with ⅓ water.

Pumpkin and squash: If you think carrots are good, take a look at the health benefits of pumpkins, which have FOUR TIMES more betacarotene than carrots. Pumpkin seed oil, which you can now buy in supermarkets as well as health stores in the UK, is a fabulous source of zinc – low levels of which have been implicated in hyperactivity and related disorders (see page 22). The seeds are also rich in the essential fatty acids that support brain development and the nervous system. Squash is not only delicious roasted but will help protect the lungs from environmental pollutants, so it is a good choice for asthmatics and kids recovering from bronchitis and other respiratory infections. It is an important food for families living in towns and cities and for children exposed to cigarette smoke.

Sweet potatoes: A good source of vitamin A and even better for eye health and night vision than carrots. Sweet potatoes also provide vitamin E, which is so important to fertility that its original name, tocopherol, is Greek for 'to bring forth children'. It protects the fatty acids that make up cell membranes from attack by free-radical molecules and is synergistic with selenium (see page 85). Bake sweet potatoes to provide more than half the daily potassium children need and use this nutritionally power-packed dish to stave off hunger pangs as part of a healthy weight management programme.

Swede: This is one of the powerful cancer-fighting brassicas, otherwise known as cruciferous vegetables. What this means is that there's much more to the humble swede than meets the eye. An excellent source of fibre, vitamin C, folate and potassium, there is evidence, according to the World Cancer Research Fund, that brassicas are the foods which, specifically, decrease the risk of cancers of the colon, rectum and thyroid in adult life. The cruciferous vegetables all contain indoles – chemicals that deactivate potent oestrogens that could otherwise trigger tumour growth in oestrogen-sensitive cells (e.g. breast tissue). The trouble with swede is that most kids hate it. Clever cooks can disguise the strong taste by mixing with a little apple sauce.

Oranges: Most people think of oranges only as a source of immune-boosting vitamin C but they also provide folacin or folic acid, which plays a role in the formation of oxygen-carrying red blood cells. Oranges also supply pectin, a soluble fibre which slows down food absorption after meals and removes unwanted toxins. Oranges can protect against cancer too, thanks to oils found in the peel. We often add grated orange peel to a simple dish of cauliflower cheese. Delicious! Watch out though for oranges that have been picked green, sprayed with red dye to make them appear ripe and then waxed to give them that glorious colour. The citric acid in green oranges has not had time to convert to fructose and they have a very low vitamin C content. You won't be able to tell just by looking, so to be sure, buy organic.

Mangoes: Mangoes provide insoluble fibre, which used to be called, somewhat less charmingly, dietary roughage. Unlike soluble fibres, which absorb water in the intestinal tract to swell to as much as ten times their weight, forming a gel that then slows down the passage of food in the gut, insoluble fibres pass through without absorption and thus have a cleansing action on the colon. A medium-sized mango provides a staggering 7g of dietary fibre. As well as providing a healthy form of carbohydrate for energy, you would also be hard-pressed to find another fruit with as much immune-boosting vitamin A, which can play a key role in the battle against teen acne (see page 289). This nutrient also promotes healthy growth of skin, hair, teeth and gums.

Apricots: Fresh apricots are a staple of the diet of the remote Hunza people who live in Kashmir, and are said to be one reason why this tribe is famous for living so long and never suffering from degenerative diseases like cancer. The cancer-preventing properties of the apricot lie in its betacarotene content – just three small, fresh apricots provide more than half the recommended daily dose of this important nutrient, as well as over a third of the amount of iron children under ten need to eat each day. They also provide potassium, which keeps the heart healthy, and magnesium which works with calcium to keep bones strong. Betacarotene can also be converted in the body into vitamin A which boosts the immune system by increasing the number of T-cells, the first line of defence against infection. Vitamin A is also important for good skin, which is why apricots often feature in natural cosmetics.

Fat-free and with no sodium, dried apricots, which are less expensive, have the nutritional edge over fresh ones because they are proportionally even higher in fibre. However, sulphites are often added during the drying process to maintain colour and preserve the betacarotene content, which can be a problem for asthmatics and other allergy sufferers. So check on the pack to make sure you are buying a sulphite-free brand.

Papaya: Rich in the digestive enzyme papain, which helps break down undigested protein and which is used by the food industry to tenderize meat, papaya is also employed in Traditional Chinese Medicine (TCM) to relieve children's coughs. Thanks to its action on protein, it can break down plaque deposits on teeth to help prevent decay and it will eliminate excess mucus and so help clear runny noses. It also has a strong vermicidal action, meaning that it is useful in preventing intestinal worms. Papaya also contains a substance called carpaine – one of the phytochemicals in plants that researchers now believe to be crucial in protecting the body from cancer.

Yellow Foods

Sweetcorn: As a good source of protein and vitamin B1, which works in the body to break down carbohydrates and convert them to that all-important body fuel, glucose, sweetcorn is important for the production of energy. And since ham and pork are more obvious sources of this same nutrient (vitamin B1), corn-on-the-cob or maize is a welcome sub-stitute in the vegetarian kitchen. Better still, kids love it. Beware the tinned versions, though – these contain five times more natural sugar than fresh corn and lots of unhealthy salt. Fresh corn was always traditionally cooked with lime to boost otherwise low niacin (vitamin B3) levels. Sweetcorn also promotes healthy growth.

Chickpeas: If you are cooking your own, soak overnight and then cook slowly using four parts water to one part beans to retain the shape. Drop a strip of kombu seaweed into the pan to improve digestibility. This will also help reduce gas. Drain and blend with olive oil, sesame seeds (which are a fantastic source of health-promoting essential fatty acids) and garlic for a delicious homemade hummus (see page 220). Chickpeas provide some calcium to growing kids (150mg per 100g/3½oz serving), and are also a rich source of complex car-bohydrates and so can help maintain even blood sugar levels and mood. Chickpeas are also one of the best legume sources of iron, which helps prevent tiredness and promotes healthy growth in children. They contain substances called protease inhibitors, too, which have been shown to prevent the conversion of normal cells into malignant ones in the early stages of cancer.

Chicory: The Americans call this Belgian endive. The slender, long, blanched young leaves are best eaten raw in a salad where they will provide a good dose of vitamins A and C, plus the all-important minerals calcium and iron. An excellent liver tonic, chicory can also help break down milk particles and so can be useful for those with developing or transient lactose intolerance (see page 349). Used in TCM as a cleansing tea for treating obesity and candida overgrowth (thrush), chicory root is often dried and ground to make a coffee substitute. It tastes OK but, to my mind, nothing like the real thing. The colour of the leaves can range from yellow to green and the plant is also a good source of heart-protecting folic acid, which also plays a key role in producing the genetic material that codes all the body's cells.

Lentils: Rich in isoflavones – cancer-protecting phytochemicals which prevent the growth of oestrogen-dependent tumours – lentils are a good source of protein and make up the perfect meal when served with rice. They are one of the best sources of genistein – the best-known of the isoflavones, which has been shown to kill off leukaemia cells in mice. Lentils also provide both types of fibre – soluble to slow down the passage of food through the gut and maximize absorption of nutrients, and insoluble to keep the colon cleansed. A member of the pea family, lentils are also rich in iron, potassium and copper. The latter is synergistic with vitamin C and so eating lentils can also help the body fight off colds and cope better with stress by enhancing the action of vitamin C. The body also needs copper to help convert iron supplies to oxygen-carrying haemoglobin. Lentils can help keep blood sugar levels under control and should be served once or twice a week.

Bananas: These strengthen the stomach lining, help lower blood cholesterol levels and have a natural antibiotic action to help protect children from infections. An almost perfect 'fast-food', a medium-sized banana provides more than half the recommended nutritional intake (RNI) of potassium for kids, which is essential for normal blood pressure and a healthy heart. It also provides a good dose of vitamin B6 which helps regulate hormones, making it useful in relieving the symptoms of PMT. Teenage girls who are taking the contraceptive pill should make a point of eating a banana a day to bolster levels of B6.

Bananas also act as a natural probiotic in the body (see page 95) to build and support higher levels of the good bacteria that promote healthy digestion and lower levels of those more harmful pathogens that can disrupt digestion. For maximum probiotic impact, serve bananas with a live, plain yoghurt. Bananas are also a good natural source of folic acid, which is important for the formation of red blood cells and can help keep DNA healthy.

Pineapples: These are a brilliant source of bromelain – the anti-inflammatory enzyme which works to soothe inflammation in the body, especially in the digestive tract. They also contain manganese, which is key to those enzymes that metabolize protein and carbohydrates, and so, again, are a good digestive aid. Bromelain can also enhance the action of antibiotics, making pineapple a good supporting food during conventional treatment for infection. That said, it can promote the production of mucus and so is not good for kids with runny noses or colds. Only buy the very ripe fruit since the acidic juice of underripe pineapples can damage teeth. Pineapple juice is a good source of vitamin C and the bromelain content can help reduce bruising.

Nectarines/Peaches: Nectarines are rich in antioxidants that help prevent the breakdown of essential fats, making them, indirectly, a good brain food. As well as providing magnesium, which is important for healthy muscles, they contain some potassium for the heart. All the yellow and orange fruits are rich in cancer-fighting carotenoids. Low on calories and high on sweet taste, these are a good fruit for those trying to control weight. Gently cook and purée peaches to soothe stomach upsets, including diarrhoea.

Lemons: Lemons can help promote weight loss – just one a day will help as part of a slim-down programme – because they help decongest the liver and speed up the digestion of fats and proteins. Lemon can boost the absorption of important minerals in the body and works internally to kill off those bad bacteria which disrupt digestion and cause bad breath. In Chinese medicine, lemons are said to calm the nerves and the mind. They also help relieve indigestion, gas and runny noses. Scientists have now found a substance called limonene in lemons. This has been shown not only to slow down the rate of cancer growths in animals but to shrink existing tumours. The best way to help children benefit from these and other health properties is to make and serve a true lemon barley water (see page 222). And since lemon juice works to enhance the flavour of other foods, keep half a lemon handy to squeeze over whatever dishes you are cooking. In winter, lemon juice helps extract the nutrients from the meats and vegetables you may be using to make healthy broths. In the summer, squeeze a little juice over salad leaves and add to homemade nut oils as dressings. If serving meat, marinade first in lemon juice to improve its digestibility.

Green Foods

Broccoli: If your kids eat no other vegetable all week, try to sneak broccoli onto their dinner plates. In fact, the more broccoli you can get them to eat, the better. Broccoli contains indoles which can protect against cell damage and cancers, monoterpenes which are antioxidants and sulphoraphane which supports the work of enzymes that stop carcinogens from damaging healthy cells. Broccoli helps the body make energy by providing vitamin B2 (riboflavin). It is also an excellent source of vitamin A, vitamin C, betacarotene and folic acid, which helps make red blood cells and DNA. Broccoli also provides vitamin K, without which no amount of calcium will give your child strong bones (see page 243) since this often overlooked vitamin is crucial for the absorption of calcium. Broccoli contains chromium, the trace mineral that works with insulin to regulate blood sugar levels, and selenium, the powerful anti-oxidant that is a major free-radical scavenger in the body. No wonder then that vegetarians, who eat lots of brassicas, are three times less likely to have a heart attack or a stroke in later life than meat eaters. Because they eat more healthy fruit and vegetables they also have a 40 per cent lower incidence of cancer and are less likely to suffer from arthritis, obesity, diet-related diabetes, constipation, gallstones, hypertension and many other ailments.

Spinach: It may have given Popeye his muscles but spinach has another more important job – it can lower levels of a substance called homo-cysteine, which could otherwise cause heart problems in later life. Homocysteine is a normal blood protein but high levels in adults have been found to be linked with higher risks of heart disease and stroke. In fact, homocysteine is now thought to be 40 times more accurate as an indicator of this risk than cholesterol. Spinach is also an excellent source of vitamin A and it provides calcium for building strong bones and teeth. That said, the oxalic acid present in the leaves can hamper the absorp-tion of calcium in the body so do not rely on spinach solely to meet the RNI. Spinach also works in the body to keep hormones balanced, mak-ing it an excellent superfood for teens (and mums) suffering from PMT or bad mood swings. It provides lutein, the hot new supplement that IT wizards take to protect eyesight. In Chinese medicine, spinach is said to have a 'sliding' action. If you can't guess what this means – it is a gentle laxative used to treat constipation.

Avocado: A superfood star no less. Providing the perfect ratio of fat, protein and carbohydrate all in one food, avocados are also rich in copper, which will ward off stress-induced headaches at homework- and exam-time. Technically a fruit but treated as a vegetable, the avocado is a natural antioxidant. It contains glutathione which blocks thirty different carcinogens and, in test-tube experiments, it has been shown to contain agents that can stop the AIDS virus from developing. The avocado pulp has both antibacterial and antifungal actions to boost resistance to disease and it also contains fluorine, another substance which helps keep the immune system healthy. Avocados are also an excellent source of the amino acid choline (also known as lecithin) which prevents liver overload, boosts memory and will help maintain an even distribution of body weight.

Peas: These little energy-bombs contain vitamin B1 (thiamine) which the body uses to convert the carbohydrates in food into energy; plus pantothenic acid, a member of the B-complex family, which helps convert other nutrients to energy too. Peas are also an excellent source of fibre and iron, and they provide manganese which activates those enzymes needed to properly use vitamin C and which plays a key role in bone growth. Researchers have found a link between eating peas and low rates of appendicitis, leading them to conclude that these vegetables must contain some agent that can suppress the bacteria that would otherwise cause this infection in the appendicular wall. Peas are high in fibre – as high as kidney beans – and low in fat, making them useful in the battle of bulging weight. And for revising schoolkids, the manganese also helps sharpen the brain.

Apples: Cut an apple in half crossways and you'll see a five-pointed star in the centre. An ancient symbol of everlasting life, it may not be the most exotic fruit you can get your hands on but it's certainly one of the most beneficial. New research has just shown that eating an apple a day can protect the lungs from toxins, including cigarette smoke. This is thanks to that brilliant bioflavonoid – quercetin. Chinese researchers at the Beijing Institute of Cancer Research, for instance, found that families eating regular amounts of quercetin in their food were 20 per cent less likely to get cancer.

Pears: A good source of cellulose fibre and lignin – a type of fibre that the good bacteria in the gut convert to cancer-fighting compounds. The high non-soluble-fibre content of pears makes them an excellent natural laxative. Purée (complete with peel) for youngsters suffering from constipation, and juice to benefit from the potassium, folic acid and vitamin C content.

Kiwi: Hard to believe but those dinky little kiwi fruits contain more immune-strengthening vitamin C than oranges. Now grown all over the world, including here, but originally native to East Asia, just one average-size kiwi has a staggering 120 per cent of the adult RNI. Low in calories – just 45 calories per fruit – kiwi, which is also known as Chinese gooseberry, can help maintain optimum weight by satisfying sweet cravings without piling on the calories. We make eating kiwi fun either at breakfast or as a dessert by serving it in an eggcup, slicing off the top and going to work on it in the same way as you would eat a boiled egg.

Limes: Used more as an accessory ingredient to enhance flavouring, limes are high in the anti-inflammatory bioflavonoids that work with vitamin C in the body to build resistance to disease. They also contain psoralens – compounds which make the skin more sensitive to sunlight and are relevant to children since synthetic forms are used to treat common skin complaints such as psoriasis (see page 365), which always improves when the skin is exposed to sunshine. Like lemons, limes have a strong antibacterial action and so can help stop runny noses and hacking coughs. For homemade lemon and lime syrup, see page 195.

Blue, Black and Purple Foods

Red cabbage: All cabbages are another excellent source of the cancer-preventing phytochemicals, a fact which first came to light when researchers started to study the Asian diet to work out why, although the incidence of some cancers was the same as in the West, deaths were much lower. What they found was a diet rich in phytochemicals, which they concluded must be the protective factor. The specific phyto-chemical in cabbage is called sulphoraphane. In laboratory trials, it has been shown to stop animals from developing breast and other cancers. Sulphoraphane is not destroyed by heat or cooking and is said to confer its anti-cancer action by destroying carcinogens in the stomach before they get a chance to cause damage. It also acts to stop cells which have taken some steps towards becoming cancerous from multiplying to form tumours. A second phytochemical found in cabbage is phenylethyl isothiocyanate (PEITC), which has now been shown to protect from lung cancer mice that were exposed to smoke.

Aubergines: Rich in the antioxidant monoterpenes, which protect tissues from free-radical damage, aubergines are a member of the Solanacae family, which includes peppers and tomatoes. In animal stud-ies, rabbits fed aubergine were protected against the formation of plaque in the arteries, even when fed a high-cholesterol diet. What happens is that the active ingredients in the vegetable bind with cholesterol from the diet in the intestinal tract, thereby preventing it from entering the bloodstream. A rich source of health-promoting bioflavonoids, aubergines guzzle up oil if fried. Better then to slice, drizzle a little oil over each circle and oven-bake on a flat tin.

Nori seaweed: Rich in fibre, low in fat and an excellent source of dietary iodine which regulates metabolism, nori also provides vitamin A, which maintains healthy skin and membranes. It can help reduce phlegm during a cold, will keep cholesterol levels down and is the most easily digested of all the sea greens. As well as making other foods more tasty, sea greens, including nori, work to release the nutritional benefits of the foods they are cooked with. They are traditionally used to flavour and tenderize other foods but also have incredible health properties in their own right. They all, for example, have cancer-fighting properties. They can help boost the immune system, deactivate the yeasts that cause common conditions such as thrush, and boost energy levels in the body by supporting the work of the thyroid gland. Sea greens are also a good source of vitamin B12, which long-term vegetarians often lack since meat is its usual dietary source. This nutrient is also known as the 'red vitamin' and is needed to make red blood cells. Nori contains more vitamin C than oranges and is easy to use. Delicious roasted and then flaked into salads, buy it from your supermarket or health store and use in soups and to make simple sushi too (see page 229).

Aduki beans: The quickest of the beans to cook, the lowest in calories and the highest in nutritional content – what more could a busy mum ask for? Aduki beans help detoxify the body and, like all beans, are a good source of folic acid, which is involved in making red blood cells. They also provide magnesium and copper, both of which the body needs to utilize vitamin C and calcium. Beans also provide zinc, which plays a key role in cell division and repair, making it an important immune-boosting and wound-healing nutrient. Beans are not only nutritious – they provide as much protein, pound for pound, as meat – but have a long shelf-life and are cheap. Beans on wholemeal toast, for example, is an excellent, healthy and balanced dish. For a simple Boston Baked Beans recipe, see page 219.

Blueberries: High in pectin – the soluble form of fibre that can help keep cholesterol levels low – and rich in vitamin C, blueberries contain active compounds called anthocyanosides which have an antibacterial action and so help build resistance to infection. Traditionally, blueberries have been used to treat diarrhoea and help control 'the runs'.

Blueberries are high in manganese, which has tissue-protecting antioxidant properties and is crucial for the production of the sex hormones. Blueberries also provide silicon for healthy tissues, iron for building healthy blood and substances which act as natural aspirins for pain relief.

Blackberries: Closely related to the raspberry and high in fibre, potassium, vitamin C and vitamin E, blackberries also contain natural chemicals called anthicyanidins which have powerful anti-inflammatory properties. They help prevent the destruction of collagen and also neutralize excess acidity in the body to relieve joint pains and aches. Blackberries also build the blood and so help prevent anaemia. Animal studies show how blackberries can help lower blood sugar levels, which is useful in preventing mood swings. For teen girls, blackberry tea (made from the leaves or roots) can help relieve menstrual cramping. Use this same tea to relieve sore throats and diarrhoea in younger children and to help clear urinary tract infections.

Figs: A fantastic digestive aid, figs are a good source of fibre, fruit sugars, folate, potassium, calcium, phosphorus, iron, copper, manganese and zinc – all nutrients which help maintain the normal chemical balance of the body and are essential for building strong bones. A sweet and delicious high energy snack, fresh figs are a perfect mid-morning treat for growing kids. Sadly, the fresh figs on sale in the UK bear no comparison to their lush Mediterranean cousins so I tend to use dried figs instead. Figs have been hailed as cancer-fighters containing properties that help shrink tumours, and the juice will clear intestinal parasite infections.

Purple grapes: There's a good reason for taking grapes to people recovering in hospital – they have long been associated with convalescence and detoxification and can help relieve a wide range of ailments from teen skin disorders to urinary infections. Grapes will help rebuild strength and banish fatigue and so are an excellent energy snack for children. All the darker varieties help build blood and ward off anaemia. Grape juice can help combat fevers in childhood and will also kick-start a sluggish digestion. In short, grapes have a cleansing effect on all the body's systems and in test-tube studies have been shown to have both antiviral and antibacterial properties. Red grapes have strong anticancer properties, are high in anti-inflammatory quercetin and can help lower blood cholesterol levels.

The Rainbow Fruit and Vegetables Food Chart

Laminated to protect it from splashes when you pin it next to the cooker, this is a simple but brilliant guide to the most important foods, charting their health benefits by colour. Simply choose your power animal stickers and aim to eat one fruit or vegetable from each of the five different colour zones every day. Make it a family contest and choose your own prize! Available by mail order only from **Stewart Distribution**, it costs £9.95 and includes enough reusable stickers for a family of five. To preview, check out the website, www.lemonburst.net. To mail-order, call 01273 625988.

Rainbow Recipes

Here are some child-friendly easy-peasy recipes to make with the kids. We've used lots of the Rainbow foods so the whole family can enjoy all the health benefits you've been reading about. In all these recipes a tablespoon (tbs) is the equivalent of 15ml.

Farmer's Market No. I Tomato Sauce

Makes about 450ml/¾ pint and easily converts to a homemade healthy pizza sauce (see page 215)

5 fresh tomatoes (about 450g/1lb) or a 400g tin chopped peeled tomatoes

6 tablespoons olive oil

I medium red pepper

4 shallots, finely chopped

I½ tsp chopped fresh thyme or half the amount dried thyme, crumbled

3 celery stalks with leaves, chopped (optional)

½ teaspoon freshly ground pepper

150g/5oz parsley, chopped

salt to taste

What you do

1) Roast the fresh tomatoes in a tablespoon of the olive oil and then remove the skins. Roast the red pepper in the same way, cool, skin, deseed and dice. Heat the remaining oil in a frying pan and add the shallots. Cook, stirring, for 1 minute. Add the thyme, tomatoes, red pepper, celery and pepper and simmer for 20 minutes. Add parsley, and salt to taste.

2) Spoon the hot sauce into small sterilized bottles or jars, leaving 3mm/⅛in of headspace. Close the jars, cool and store in the fridge. Use within three months.

Five-star Tip

For a healthy pizza sauce, substitute basil for the parsley and add oregano with the thyme. Lemon juice is a great way to bring out the flavours hidden in the sauce and you can coax them out by adding the juice of half a lemon for the last five minutes of cooking. An interesting variation to the No. 1 Tomato Sauce is to omit the red pepper and add 200g/7oz of grated butternut squash, which melts into the sauce and gives a wonderful sweet flavour in contrast to the sharpness of the lemon.

Farmer's Market No. 2 Tomato Ketchup

Makes about 350ml/12fl oz

3 medium onions, finely chopped

1 small clove garlic, finely chopped

2 tbs olive oil

2 sweet red peppers roasted in olive oil, peeled, deseeded and chopped
    (try to retain the juice)

double portion of Farmer's Market No. 1 Tomato Sauce (900ml/1½ pints)

spice bag made up of a 5cm/2in stick of cinnamon, 1 tsp peppercorns,
    1 tsp cloves, 1 tsp whole all-spice, 1 tsp celery seed

120g/4oz brown sugar (preferably demerara)

250ml/½ pint rice wine vinegar

juice of a lemon

1 tsp salt

2 tsp paprika

¼ tsp cayenne pepper

What you do

1) To make an authentic and unforgettable tomato ketchup start with a double portion of the No. 1 Tomato Sauce. Take a heavy-based saucepan and cook the onions and garlic in the olive oil until the onion is soft and translucent.

2) Add the red peppers and cook for another five minutes before adding the retained red pepper juice. Add the double portion of the No. 1 Tomato Sauce. When this mix comes to the boil, strain through a fine sieve and set the strained solids to one side.

3) Return the sauce to the saucepan and simmer for 30–40 minutes or until the mixture is reduced by half, stirring frequently to make sure that it does not stick or burn. Add the spice bag and the rest of the ingredients and continue to cook slowly, stirring frequently to prevent it burning or sticking, until the liquor is very thick.

4) Remove from the heat, take out the bag of spices and stir in the retained solids. Allow to cool slightly and then blend to a medium consistency. Spoon into small sterilized jars, leaving 3mm/⅛in headspace. Close the jars, cool, refrigerate and use within three months.

No-Q Pizza

Serves 2 teen piggies or 4 piglets

Who says that a take-away pizza is the only pizza treat for you, your family and friends?

1 ciabatta loaf
2 tbs olive oil
200ml/7fl oz No. 1 Tomato Sauce (page 214) prepared with basil and
  oregano rather than parsley and thyme (if the only sauce you have has

been made with parsley and thyme, don't worry, just add a tablespoon of fresh or a teaspoon of dry basil and the same of oregano to that sauce)

grated mozzarella cheese (if you don't have mozzarella cheese then you can use medium to strong cheddar instead)

What you do

1) Preheat the oven to 230°C/450°F/Gas 8. Take the ciabatta loaf and slice it open lengthwise and then across the middle into four pieces.

2) Coat a baking tray with olive oil (for the method, see Aubergine Pizza Wheels, page 226) and place each slice, crust-side up, on it. Pop into the oven for about 5 minutes until the underside begins to turn a golden brown. Remove from the oven, turn over so you now have the bread crust-side down, and then spread No. 1 Tomato Sauce evenly and generously on each slice. Scatter grated mozzarella cheese on top. Again, be generous. Now drizzle with olive oil and return the tray to the oven for about 10–15 minutes or until this topping is piping hot, crisp and golden.

*****

Five-star Tip

You can vary this dish using different toppings. Experiment with spicy sausage for meat-eating older kids, olives, anchovies or capers, and make a Turf 'n' Surf Supreme Pizza with smoked ham, mushrooms, prawns and pineapple.

Raspberry Jelly Secrets

Makes 6 individual jellies

Use agar agar (from health stores) instead of gelatin, which is made from slaughterhouse by-products. A Japanese gelatin made from seaweed, agar agar contains no calories and comes in three forms – flakes, bar form or granulated. Use two tablespoons of flakes to 900ml/1½ pints of liquid; 18cm/7in of bar to the same quantity of fluid; or one tablespoon of granulated agar agar. First, though, soak it in 250ml/½ pint of liquid before adding the remaining liquid. It thickens as it cools and is an excellent source of fibre, making this a good dish for kids suffering from constipation.

Even without refrigeration, the mixture of date and raspberry juice and agar agar will set quickly. As it cools it seals in the natural flavour and sweetness of the raspberry, yoghurt and honey hiding in the centre.

6 fresh dates (fresh is best but dried can be used)

1.5kg/3lb whole raspberries (again fresh is best but frozen can be substituted)

6 tbs Greek sheep's yoghurt

6 tbs Cretan thyme honey (or your own family's favourite)

225g/8oz agar agar (gelling agent available from health stores)

What you do

1) You need 6 cup-size jelly moulds. Place them in your freezer.

2) Boil the dates in 900ml/1½ pints of water for about 10 minutes or until the fruits have lost their shape. Drain the date juice and reserve.

3) Take 12 whole raspberries from your bowl and set aside. Place the remaining raspberries in a saucepan, add the date juice, cover the pan and bring to the boil, then simmer for 10 minutes or until the raspberries

have given up their juices. Strain the mixture and measure out 6 jelly-mouldsful of the liquid into a pan. (If necessary top up with cold water.)

4) Add the agar agar (snow-dried if available) and let it sit in the pan for 10 to 15 minutes. Then bring the pan back to the boil, lower the heat and allow to simmer for 3–4 minutes, stirring constantly, until the agar agar flakes have dissolved.

5) Take the jelly moulds from the freezer and pour about a centimetre of jelly juice into each. Swish each mould around so that the jelly juice coats the sides and place them in your fridge for 10 to 15 minutes until the juice has set. Take the moulds out and place two raspberries, a dollop of yoghurt and blob of honey into each. This is the delicious secret centre!

6) Finally, cover each of the moulds with the remaining jelly juice and place all the moulds in the fridge until you are ready. To serve, place each mould in a bowl of hot water for 10 to 15 seconds before turning the jelly out on pudding plates.

Rainbow Orange Foods

Boston Baked Beans – the Real McCoy!

Serves 6 children or a family of 5

450g/1lb dry french navy or haricot beans
1 tbs salt (preferably sea salt)
2 tsp dry mustard
2½ tbs brown sugar (preferably demerara)
2 tbs molasses or black treacle
1 medium onion, chopped
1 clove garlic, chopped

450ml/¾ pint vegetable stock

450ml/¾ pint **Farmer's Market No. I Tomato Sauce (page 214)**

juice of I lemon

sea salt and black pepper to taste

Worcestershire sauce, optional

What you do

1) Wash the beans and either soak overnight or, if pressed for time, cheat by putting the beans in a pot, cover with three times the volume of water and bring to the boil. Remove from the heat, keep covered and leave standing for an hour. Drain the beans and place in a large oven-proof casserole and cover with water. Add the salt and bring to a rapid boil for ten minutes, then simmer, covered, for 45 minutes on the hob.

2) Drain the cooked beans and return to the casserole with the remaining ingredients. Mix thoroughly, season with salt and pepper, cover and bake in the oven at 150°C/300°F/Gas 2 for 4 hours, until the beans are tender. Check and stir the beans occasionally; where necessary add water.

3) Taste and adjust seasoning if necessary before serving. For more oomph, add two or three tablespoons of Worcestershire sauce during baking.

Rainbow Yellow Foods

Chunky Chickpea Hummus

Serves 6 children or a family of 4

225g/8oz tin organic chickpeas, drained

juice of I fresh lemon

1 tbs tahini (sesame seed paste)

4 tbs Greek sheep's yoghurt

3 tbs olive oil (Greek if available)

1 clove garlic

sea salt and black pepper to taste

to serve: olive oil, parsley or coriander, lemon wedges, pitta or ciabatta
   bread (see recipe)

What you do

1) Reserve ¼ of the chickpeas and ½ the lemon juice. Place all the remaining ingredients, except the salt and pepper, into a blender and whizz until well mixed and smooth. Add the remaining chickpeas and lemon juice and blend for short bursts until the chickpeas are broken up but not ground into the mixture. Season to taste.

2) Turn out onto a serving dish, cover and place in the fridge to chill. Drizzle with olive oil and sprinkle with finely chopped parsley or coriander leaves and garnish with lemon wedges before serving with toasted pocket pitta or ciabatta bread.

3) Put 2 tablespoons of Chunky Chickpea Hummus in a small sealable bowl and pack with strips of carrot, cucumber and some cauliflower florets (plus a lemon wedge for older kids) to make a healthy lunchbox dip.

*****
Five-star Tip
As a colourful variation, add a handful of coriander leaves or a skinned and deseeded roasted red pepper to the first mixture before blending until smooth.

Declan's Homemade Lemon Barley Water

Serves 4 children or a family of 4

In the winter, everyone thinks we're mad to live so high up in the Chiltern hills where the fog can hang around for days and we never seem to get out of our wellington boots. But they're not here when the sun does shine and Declan brings out his home-made lemon barley water so we can all sit on the deck (the only 'townie' bit of the garden), smell the herbs from my meditation garden and watch the sun set. Sheer bliss.

50g/2oz pearl barley
50g/2oz soft brown sugar
juice of 2 large or 3 small fresh lemons

What you do

1) Pour the pearl barley into a saucepan. Add water until it just covers the grain and bring to the boil. Drain and rinse the barley under cold water. Return the barley to the saucepan and add 600ml/1 pint of cold water and bring to the boil again. Cover and simmer for 1 hour.

2) Remove from the heat, strain the liquid into a jug or basin, stir in the sugar and cool. When the syrup is cold, add the strained lemon juice and stir the mixture. Dilute with iced filtered water to serve. The undiluted drink can be stored in the fridge in a screw-topped bottle.

*****

Five-star Tip

You can also use this recipe to make orange, grapefruit or lime barley water by substituting these fruits for the lemons. To give the orange barley water bite, use two oranges and a lemon for enhanced fruity flavouring.

Captain Hook's Hand of Cod with Green Kiwi and Ruby Salsa

Serves 4 children or a family of 4

Forget boring old fish fingers. This is a spooky recipe which was found in an old shipwreck by an intrepid cabin boy who looked a lot like Peter Pan. The golden pieces of fresh cod are treasure enough, but when dressed with the chunks of emerald (kiwi) in the ruby-coloured salsa they make a meal fit for pirates.

I plump fillet of cod (get the fishmonger to bone and skin it)

3 tbs flour

3 tbs breadcrumbs

I egg

salt and pepper to taste

sunflower or vegetable oil

I small cube dry bread

I recipe quantity Bright Green Kiwi and Ruby Salsa (page 224)

What you do

1) Take the fillet of cod and place it on a chopping board with the thinner end furthest from you. Cut the last third of the fillet off, cut this into four equal lengths to make the Hand of Cod and move to one side.

2) Take the remaining large piece of cod and cut four lengthwise strips. These longer strips will look like four fingers. Place these on a long dish or tray. Use three of the other pieces of cod to form the palm at the end of the fingers of cod and arrange the last piece of cod where a thumb should be. This is the way that you will arrange the eight pieces of cod when you present them at the table.

3) Now take two plates and a bowl. Put the flour on one plate and breadcrumbs on the other. Break and beat the egg in the bowl and season with salt and pepper. Clean and dry your hands, then, taking each piece of cod, dip and coat it first in the flour, then in the beaten egg and lastly in the breadcrumbs. Then place each piece of cod hand back on the serving dish in its proper place. Now wash your hands again.

4) Half fill a frying pan with sunflower oil and put over a high heat. Place a piece of dry bread in the frying pan. When the bread starts to fizzle you'll know the oil is at the right temperature to start cooking the fish.

5) Take the four fingers from the cod arrangement and, using tongs or a fish slice, gently drop them into the oil. Let the fingers bubble and fizz for a minute or two and then check underneath one using a fish slice. When the bottom side has turned a golden brown, turn all the fingers over and cook on the other side until golden brown.

6) Take the fingers out of the frying pan and place on a serving plate covered with a sheet of kitchen paper. Cover with a saucepan lid to keep hot and repeat this cooking process with the other pieces of cod. When all the pieces of fish have been cooked, rearrange these golden pieces of cod into Captain Hook's Lonely Hand. Heap the emeralds of the Kiwi Salsa onto the fingers and into the palm and serve.

Bright Green Kiwi and Ruby Salsa

Serves 4

1 shallot, chopped

1 tbs olive oil

juice from half a lime

1 kiwi fruit, peeled

1 tbs Farmer's Market No. 1 Tomato Sauce (page 214)

1 tsp honey
salt and pepper to taste

What you do

1) Sweat the shallot in the olive oil. Take off the heat to cool and add the lime juice. Chop the kiwi fruit into fine cubes and add to the shallot and lime mixture, then add the Farmer's Market No. 1 Tomato Sauce together with the honey and season with salt and pepper to taste.

2) Place this mix into a serving dish and leave in the fridge for an hour or so to draw out the flavours. Serve with Captain Hook's Hand of Cod (page 223).

Avocado and Lime Ice Cream Footballs

Serves a family of 5

Vitamins A, C and E are the three most powerful antioxidants, which help the body fight stress. Besides these, this dish also provides selenium, which enhances the action of vitamin E in the body and is crucial for developing reproductive organs and for teen health.

4 egg yolks
300ml/½pt whipping cream
120g/4oz granulated sugar
2 ripe avocados
grated rind and juice of 2 limes
2 egg whites
a twist of lime, a sprig of mint and a few shelled pistachio nuts* to serve

*Forget the nuts if there is any underlying allergy.

What you do

1) Beat the egg yolks. In a saucepan, heat the cream with the sugar and stir well, until dissolved. Bring to a gentle boil and, as the cream rises to the top of the pan, remove from the heat. Gently pour the egg yolks into the scalded cream from a great height to stop curdling. Whisk constantly. Transfer to a bowl. Allow to cool, stirring occasionally, then chill in the fridge.

2) Peel and mash the avocados until smooth. Beat into the chilled egg and cream custard with the lime rind and juice. Check for sweetness and add extra sugar if it tastes a bit bland. Ice cream should be very sweet as it loses some flavour when ice-cold.

3) Pour this mixture into a freezerproof container with a lid and freeze until slushy. Remove from the freezer and whisk well to prevent large ice crystals from forming. Whisk the egg whites until they form peaks and then fold into the ice cream mixture. Return to the freezer and leave until set. Remove every half an hour to whisk again and prevent ice crystals.

4) Remove the ice cream from the freezer 10 minutes before you want to serve. Use a melon baller to make little individual footballs and serve for half-time with a twist of lime, a sprig of mint (which is tastier than grass) and a scattering of potassium-rich shelled pistachio nuts.

Rainbow Blue, Black or Purple Foods

Aubergine Pizza Wheels

Makes 6 wheels – enough for a lorry or 3 hungry children, or a starter for a family of 6

225g/8oz aubergine
salt

I ball of mozzarella cheese

I tbs olive oil

6 tbs Farmer's Market No. I Tomato Sauce (page 214)

fresh bread to serve

What you do

1) Take the aubergine and slice it into six pieces about 1cm/½in thick. Sprinkle some salt across the top of each of the slices and leave for about 30 minutes. (For the school swots among you, this is called degorging the aubergine, which has nothing to do with being sick!)

2) While you wait, take the ball of mozzarella cheese and slice into six circles. Put to one side. Preheat the oven to 200°C/400°F/Gas 6.

3) After about 25 minutes, take a medium-sized saucepan, half fill with filtered water, put a steamer into it and bring to the boil.

4) When the 30 minutes are up, rinse the aubergine slices under running cold water and pat dry with kitchen paper or a clean drying towel. Place the dry slices in the steamer on the heat, cover with a lid and leave to steam for 10 minutes.

5) Remove the pan from the heat. Take a baking tray and drizzle the olive oil onto it (tip from side to side for the oil to cover the entire surface). Place the tray beside the saucepan and transfer the steamed slices of aubergine onto the baking tray using a spoon underneath and a fork above each slice.

6) Put a tablespoonful of No. I Tomato Sauce on each aubergine wheel, and smear all over, then place a slice of mozzarella cheese on top. Pop the tray into the hot oven. Leave for 15 minutes, checking occasionally.

7) When the top of the cheese has turned golden brown, the wheels are done and ready to serve with a hunk of fresh bread to mop up all the tasty juices that will escape.

Figgy Piggy Muffins

Makes 12 bite-size muffins

This recipe is so quick you can make it while the breakfast tea or coffee is brewing, pop up for your shower and come down to serve these delicious mini muffins for breakfast. Alternatively, pack them in the kids' lunchboxes.

4 fresh figs or 8 dried figs, roughly chopped

5 cardamom pods

140g/5oz self-raising flour, sifted

60g/2oz caster sugar

1 egg, beaten

3 tbs sunflower oil

3 tbs milk

grated zest of 1 lemon

What you do

1) Preheat the oven to 180°C/350°F/Gas 4. If using dried figs, soak them in hot water for 5 minutes. Pop the cardamom pods in a mortar. Briefly grind them with a pestle to break up the pods. Remove the pieces of pod and grind the little black seeds.

2) Sift the flour into a large mixing bowl and add the ground cardamom seeds and the caster sugar. Stir and then make a well in the centre of this dry mix. Pour in the beaten egg, oil and milk. Stir the mixture thoroughly but gently.

3) Mix the figs with the lemon zest, stir into the mixture in the bowl and then spoon into paper cases set in a muffin tray. Bake in the oven for 20–25 minutes or until well risen and golden brown on top. Serve warm for breakfast, or cool on a wire baking rack and pack for lunch.

Simple Ten-Step Sushi
(yes, really, it's simple and look, no raw fish!)

Makes 24 slices at 1cm/½in thick, which is enough for 4 lunches or appetizers for a family of 6

Sushi is not only trendy, it's healthy too. I've yet to meet a kid who doesn't like it! The original fast food, the idea is that it's made on street corners while you, the customer, stand there ordering the delicacies you fancy. In Japan, sushi chefs serve a long apprenticeship. However, this Rainbow recipe for a dead simple sushi roll could not be easier. It's worth persevering with the rolling technique, which can take a few attempts to perfect.

You'll need a few pieces of kit to get going – most important, of course, is the bamboo rolling mat, which you can now buy in most good cookery shops and department stores. If you get hooked, you can also invest in a wooden rice tub (which is porous enough to absorb the excess moisture from the sushi rice as it cools) and a wooden rice paddle to spread the cooled rice on your rolling mat.

Finally, every sushi chef worth his or her salt uses a large fan to cool the cooked sushi rice and cut down the preparation time. You can use a foldaway fan or even a strong cardboard sheet to the same effect. When you really get into sushi-making, you could sensibly invest in an electric fan to speed up the entire process. Sushi rice is a special short grain, glutinous rice which you can now buy in supermarkets here.

200g/7oz sushi rice
1 chicken breast
grated fresh ginger
3 tbs milk
2 tbs Japanese rice vinegar
1½ tbs sugar

1 tbs salt

1 medium carrot, peeled

5cm/2in length cucumber

½ avocado

2 finger dabs Japanese horseradish, known as wasabi

1 tbs soy sauce

3 sheets of nori (Japanese seaweed which is black/green in colour)

leaves or garden fronds to garnish

pickled ginger and Japanese soy sauce to serve

What you do

1) Preheat the oven to medium. Take the sushi rice and rinse in cold water until the water runs clear. Then put the rice in a saucepan with 300ml/½pint of water. Cover with a tight-fitting lid and bring to the boil. Reduce the heat and simmer for about five minutes and then reduce the heat still further to steam the rice for another 12–15 minutes.

2) While the rice is steaming, take the chicken breast and place on a sheet of aluminium foil that is big enough to fold and twist into a cooking parcel. Add some grated fresh ginger and the milk and poach on a tray in the medium oven.

3) Take another saucepan and pour the rice vinegar, sugar and salt into it. Bring to the boil and stir. When the sugar and the salt have dissolved take the pan off the heat and allow to cool. Now it should be time to take the chicken breast out of the oven and to take the steaming rice off the heat. Allow the rice to stand for a further 15 minutes.

4) While the rice is standing, make thin matchsticks of the carrot, cucumber and avocado. Put on a dish to one side. Take the chicken breast, cut it lengthwise into strips and set aside. Take the 2 finger dabs of wasabi (hot horseradish sauce) and mix it in a dish with the soy sauce. Set aside.

5) Now empty the cooked rice into a shallow dish and gently separate the grains of rice with a fork, wooden spatula, or rice paddle if you have

one. Slowly add the rice vinegar mixture and draw the fork or spatula lightly through the rice so that all the grains are coated. The more care you take with this, the better your sushi roll will be. Fan the mixture until it reaches room temperature and then cover with a clean cloth until you need it.

6) Take the bamboo mat and roll it open away from you. Take one sheet of nori seaweed and place it on the mat, lining up one edge of the seaweed with the edge of the mat that is closest to you. Take a third of the vinegared rice and gently spread over the sheet of seaweed in an even layer, leaving about a 2.5cm/1in strip of the seaweed visible at the side farthest from you and about a 1cm/½in strip visible at the edge closest to you.

7) Smear a fingertipful of the wasabi and soy sauce mix over the rice in a line, from left to right, about one third up from the closest edge of the seaweed sheet.

8) Next, take a third of each of the filling ingredients and lay them in horizontal strips from the left to the right edge, starting from the line of wasabi and moving away from you.

9) Once all the fillings are in place, pick up the edge of mat together with the edge of the seaweed side nearest to you in your thumbs and index fingers. Using your middle fingers to hold the mat and the filling in place, fold the mat and the sheet away from you and onto the filling. Fold the edge of the sheet of seaweed under itself and then push the bamboo mat away from you so that the seaweed and its ingredients roll up into a cylinder. While the sushi roll is contained in the mat, press downwards and then on the side of the cylinder to give the roll flat sides and bottom. Unroll the mat and leave the roll to stand under a clean drying-up cloth. Carry on to make the next two rolls.

10) To prepare the sushi slices, take a very sharp knife and dip the blade in fresh water. Without drying it, take each roll and cut it in half. Trim either end and rinse and wet the knife again. Cut each half into half again

and cut each quarter in two. Repeat with the other rolls and present the portions on a large plate decorated with green leaves or fronds from the garden. Serve with Japanese soy sauce and pickled ginger, which will be available in any good supermarket or health food store.

*****
Five-star Tip
Invest in a sushi starter kit (£14.99 from Simply Sushi on 07971 412305) and let the kids have a go! At just 300 calories for a six-piece sushi lunchbox, this is also the perfect meal for older kids and mums or dads watching their weight.

PART FOUR

Your Changing Child

Understanding the changes,
and how natural remedies help

Introduction

American doctors have now confirmed it is safe to give children age-appropriate doses of the supplements that have taken the ever-sickening developed world by storm in the last decade. But what we have to recognize is that children's bodies are simply not the same as ours. The child's heart, for instance, beats harder and faster, which may seem alarming but is entirely normal. The digestive system does not fully develop until the age of three and in infancy and toddlerhood is more permeable than that of an older child. Did you know the immune system is not considered mature until the age of fourteen, by which time your child, if you vaccinate him or her, will have been deliberately 'infected' over thirty times to artificially stimulate the body's own defences? We all talk about the immune system a great deal but how many of us know anything about how it really works?

In this section, we take a look at your changing child and explore not only how what is happening on the inside will affect the way your child looks, moves and behaves, but also how you can use natural medicine to support these developing systems, especially during times of stress. For instance, if you're dealing with a teen facing crucial exams, you might like to know about the safe supplements designed to boost short-term memory which will make all the difference to their confidence and could even make the difference between a pass or fail. All you are doing is giving nature a helping hand, or a gentle nudge.

We start the section at the beginning with the newborn brain which neuroscientists now confirm has many more latent skills than anyone ever realized. You'll find out why your toddler is going to outsmart you every time. We work our way through all the body's systems from the heart and lungs to the skeleton; from the digestive system to the complex endocrine mechanism which governs those rampaging teen hormones. You may not, for example, even notice the influence of testosterone on your male children until the teens but its presence establishes significant physical and behavioural differences between the sexes from the age of two or three.

We all now know the importance of strong bones and teeth in childhood but have you become what orthopaedic doctors and nurses call a 'semi-skimmed Muesli Mum', doing your best to get the kids to eat a healthier, low-fat diet but inadvertently putting them at risk of a calcium deficiency that could cost them dear in later life? If the answer is yes, you'll be tempted to rush out now and buy calcium supplements for the whole family – but before you do, stop and read this section, which will tell you why, without another substance you've probably never even heard of, all the calcium in the world won't make a jot of difference.

Maybe you suspect your teen daughter is having unprotected sex. An unplanned teen pregnancy ought not to be your only fear. She is also at risk of being infected by a virus, some strains of which scientists now know for sure plays a pivotal role in cervical cancer. To find out how to protect her, even when you're scared it's too late (it's not), read the section on hormones.

Bulging Brains – The Mini Einstein in your Home

Sad but true, your smarty-pants child really is cleverer than you. You already know they have a mind of their own, but what a mind! In the last thirty years, researchers have made huge strides in their understanding of how the human brain works, and now, thanks to new techniques which can measure the activity and energy consumption of the brain, we know that a child of three has a brain that is *twice* as active as that of its parents. And once you understand a little more about how the brain works, you will see how you can use natural remedies to support it as it grows.

Baby Brains

A baby's brain weighs just a quarter of the weight of your brain (yours is around the same weight as a bag of sugar) yet the infant brain already has most of the neurons or nerve cells it will ever need. What increases the brain mass as your child grows is the growth of the connections between nerve cells, which enable them to 'talk' to each other. Investigations of the embryonic brain in early pregnancy show how, even at this stage, some primitive wiring between cells is already taking place. But most of the new connections take place after birth in response to new activities and experiences.

After birth, a newborn child is bombarded with sensory experience and the brain cells respond to these stimuli by firing off electrical impulses and trying to connect to nearby cells. Groups of cells send signals out in waves to try to reach other cells and those that fire at the same time are the ones that will make a connection. As neuroscientists say, cells that fire together, wire together. At first, these brain cells are promiscuous and indiscriminate, trying to connect to as many other cells as they can. When another cell responds, and does so often enough, a link or connection between the two gets laid down to form a more permanent and meaningful connection.

How it works

Nerve cells have two distinct branches to gather and send out information. The **axons** are the branches sending information out. The **dendrites** are the branches bringing information back into the cell. The aim then, for the growing brain, is for the axons of one cell to connect with the dendrites of another. This connection, when made, is called a **synapse**. The process is known as **synaptogenesis**.

Once two nerve cells have formed a synapse, the brain chemicals or **neurotransmitters**, which in effect control the whole of the rest of the body's functions, can flow between the two and the cells can 'talk' to each other.

Toddler Brains

At birth, each nerve cell in the cerebral cortex, or thinking part of the brain, has around 2,500 synapses. This figure peaks at the age of three, when it is closer to 15,000 synapses per nerve cell – many, many more than the adult brain.

New techniques, which allow neuroscientists to study living

brains, have revealed how it is not certain parts of the brain that respond to specific stimuli but certain individual cells. Some cells, for instance, respond only to faces. Some respond only to the familiar faces of parents or siblings. Some respond to particular shapes. Others only become active when a distinctive noise is heard. This sophisticated cell 'tuning' is very precise and when a cell 'sees' or 'hears' something it likes, it creates a burst of electrical activity that communicates what it has perceived to other parts of the brain. Groups of individual cells all firing in this way work like the circuits of a computer. The big difference between the workings of the brain and that of a computer, though, is that the brain keeps on rewiring itself, even after it has been turned on.

Schoolkid Brains

You may think ageing starts at around thirty but, incredibly, the human brain actually begins to slow down at around the age of nine or ten. Between then and age eighteen, the number of synapses being formed will slowly decline to the level that will be maintained in the adult brain. (Which might explain why it can be easier to outsmart your teenager than your toddler.) It is estimated that it takes a quadrillion connections, that is, 1,000 trillion, to wire an adult brain, and it is those specific patterns of connection that will define the unique individual your child will become.

Teen Brains

If you have a love-lorn teen mooching around the house, make friends with the biochemistry of that young brain. What love-lorn teens are actually suffering from is a withdrawal of phenylethylalanine – the brain chemical linked with the wonderful high of being in love. If dumped (or if the love remains unrequited), the brain stops its output of this chemical, which is derived from phenylalanine – an amino acid found in many everyday foods but especially chocolate. Other foods to help comfort the heartbroken include almonds, apples, carrots, chicken, peanuts, pineapple, eggs, tomatoes, beetroot and, somewhat unromantically, herring!

Brain Foods

The single most important nutrient for brain health and development, from conception to adulthood, is **DHA**, or **docosahexaenoic acid**. One of the hard-to-source omega-3 essential fatty acids, it cannot be made by the body (except during pregnancy) and so must come from the diet. The trouble is, it is a fragile nutrient that is easily destroyed by food processing techniques and by cooking.

The reason DHA is the most important of the brain nutrients is that it plays a key role in synaptogenesis – the formation of the synapses which allow information to travel between cells in the brain. Almost a third of the brain is believed to be made up of DHA and in animal studies, when this nutrient is removed from the diet, scientists report seriously impaired learning skills.

DHA is involved in the transmission of nerve impulses, in the formation of myelin – the protective fatty sheath that covers nerve cells to accelerate these transmissions – and in energy production. Interestingly, when it comes to optimum brain nutrition, we can learn almost everything we need to know from nature since the single best source of DHA for human infants is breastmilk.

If you have toddlers or schoolkids and want to help their brains reach and maintain their full potential, make sure you serve foods that are rich in the omega fatty acids (nuts, seeds, legumes and vegetable oils), including DHA. For these younger kids, **Omega Nutrition's Essential Balance Jnr** provides a 1:1 ratio of omega-3 and omega-6 fats and can easily be hidden in fruit juices and smoothies (see pages 188–96). Mail-order from the Nutri Centre on 020 7436 5122. (Breast-fed babies get the fatty acids they need from breastmilk. If bottle feeding, check the formula you are using is one that has been supplemented with fatty acids.)

Forget fashion accessories – your exam-crazed teen needs food ones

Accessory nutrients are those substances the body can make but not in high enough doses to give the maximum health benefits. The brain chemical **acetylcholine** – made from choline – is one of these. Secreted at the synapses where it helps transport messages between cells, depressed levels are linked to memory loss and, in adults, to conditions such as Alzheimer's disease. If you give someone a drug that blocks the action of acetylcholine in the brain, you will cause a temporary memory loss, leading researchers to conclude this nutrient must play a key role in remembering.

Choline is a member of the B-complex vitamin family and the best food sources are eggs, liver (remember how your own mother told you to eat up your liver?), soybeans, green beans, lentils and peanuts, plus cold-pressed oils such as sunflower and sesame. The normal dietary intake of choline is 300mg a day, but to boost memory researchers recommend an Optimum Nutrition Intake (ONI) of between 1g and 3g for adults. Choline may be sold as phosphatidylcholine or phosphatidylinositol. Solgar's Choline capsules are 350mg strength. 100 veggie capsules cost £9.45 from the Nutri Centre (020 7436 5122). Give teens over the age of fourteen one or two capsules daily.

Mood Boosters

Psychonutrition – the idea of using food to alter brain chemistry and mood – is both fascinating and controversial, dividing not just orthodox and alternative health practitioners but those purportedly on the same side of the divide. Scientists have now identified some forty neurotransmitters and one of the most important (and better known) of these is **serotonin**. It is linked with sleep patterns, mood and perceptions. Too little may cause sleeplessness and depression. Too much has been linked with psychosis and aggression.

The brain makes serotonin from a common amino acid called **tryptophan** which can be found in foods such as spinach, cauliflower, broccoli, cottage cheese, fennel, fish, sweet potatoes, turkey, soybeans, chicken and watercress. To enhance the transport of tryptophan across the blood–brain barrier, which allows only oxygen, glucose and a few selected nutrients to pass through, you need to step up your child's intake of carbohydrates. These cause the pancreas to make more insulin which, in turn, gets rid of other amino acids which would otherwise compete with tryptophan to reach the brain.

What to use

Tryptophan, then, is needed to make serotonin, and this is what you can buy in supplements where it is called 5-hydroxy-tryptophan or 5-HTP. **Serotone**, made by Higher Nature, is also rich in the anti-stress and oxygen-to-brain boosting B vitamins, especially B6, so this is the one I recommend for older kids at exam time. 30 capsules, which contain 100mg of tryptophan each, cost £14.80. Mail-order on 01435 882880.

Bones and Teeth

The most important mineral for strong, healthy bones is **calcium**. There is more calcium in the human body than any other mineral – about 3lb (almost 1.5kg) in an adult – and most of it is stored in the bones and teeth. Some 20 per cent of the calcium in our bones is reabsorbed and replaced every year as old bone cells break down and new ones form to keep the skeleton strong. This is an ongoing process, and what it means is that in childhood the whole skeleton is replaced once every two years (in adults, this process takes seven years). Most people assume that if you get enough calcium in the diet you will build and keep strong bones and teeth, but this is not the case. To understand why a strong skeleton needs so much more, you need to know how bone is made.

First, you need a mesh of microfibres for the calcium and magnesium minerals to cling to. This mesh, called the **osteoid**, is made up of proteins, collagen, elastin and various glucosamine polymers (which is why lots of adult supplements* for healthy joints include glucosamine). To build these proteins, the body

---

*Adult formulations, which include collagen, chondroitin and glucosamine, are not suited to kids under twelve.

needs vitamin C, vitamin B6, copper and zinc. To make glucos-amine polymers, the body needs glucosamine and manganese, and to activate the whole matrix, you need vitamin K.

Once this matrix is built and active, it is then impregnated with the calcium and magnesium salts the body uses to form solid bone. But the single most important substance the body needs to make and keep strong bones is one few people have even heard of: **ipriflavone**. This is a flavonoid and an extract of soya which has been shown in adult clinical trials to reduce bone loss and promote bone-building. Nobody has yet researched the outcome of giving ipriflavone supplements to kids so the current advice is only to do so in critical cases of bone density deficiency, and not to do so at all if there is any underlying liver complaint, since con-cerns have been raised that the soya extract could interfere with liver enzymes. What you can safely do is step up your child's intake of this important nutrient by increasing ipriflavone-rich foods in the diet, including beans (such as baked beans!) and soya products.

You can make sure your growing child is getting all these important micronutrients by combining good nutrient supple-mentation with a healthy diet. Broccoli, for instance, is a brilliant source of vitamin K. Eggs are a good source of vitamin B6. Tofu made from soya will provide ipriflavone (see Smoothies, page 195). And the oily fish such as salmon and mackerel provide the essential fatty acids that are also needed for maintaining a strong skeleton. (For details about how to safely supplement these and other nutrients, see Supplements, pages 64–95.)

One of the few supplements formulated to help strengthen the bones for kids over the age of four, **Saludynam** is a liquid calcium, magnesium, zinc and vitamin D formulation that includes herbal extracts of hibiscus flowers, chamomile, fennel and spinach. It also contains mango juice and orange juice for flavouring. It costs £7.49 for 250ml from the Nutri Centre on 020 7436 5122.

Baby Bones

Throughout childhood and adolescence, the developing skeleton changes and moulds according to the forces exerted on it by your child's muscles, other parts of the skeleton and, of course, in line with their genetic inheritance. By the end of the fourth week of life in the womb, specialized connective tissue in the region of the future skeleton is already showing signs of differentiation. Primitive cells pack together more closely and lay down a cartilage matrix that is rich in a substance called chondroitin sulphate. At six weeks, the vertebrae of the spine are forming, and by eight weeks, ossification can be seen via an ultrasound scan.

In newborns, the spine has two primary curves. By puberty, the number will have doubled to four, giving the spine its familiar S-shape curve, which it needs to support the weight of the head and upper body. If you look at your baby's head, you will see the bones of the skull are thin and the facial bones and jaw are very small, yet at birth the newborn's head is, proportionally, twice the size of that of an adult. In other words, it's big and heavy.

At four months, babies pull their head up to try to balance it on top of the spine. At eight months, they have the strength they need to sit up. By this time, you will notice one of the two secondary curves developing at the bottom or lumbar region of the spine in preparation for walking.

Toddler Bones

By the first birthday, most children are starting to stand. This demands a wide gait to balance that top-heavy skull. To achieve this, the lumbar curve now becomes more exaggerated, and the toddler will stand with its stomach sticking out. This is the only way toddlers can hold the upper part of the body and that heavy head erect, until the muscles in the back have developed enough strength to maintain a standing posture. To help strengthen the lower back, practise a little gentle yoga with children over three (see page 148).

Skeletal age in preschoolers is measured from the twenty bones in the left wrist and hand, which are then compared with a standard measurement. At this stage, girls are usually around two years ahead of boys. Although the bones of the face and jaw have grown since infancy, they are still relatively small, which is why children under seven who need medical resuscitation must be treated with a different technique than adults.

Small children also have small facial sinuses (see A–Z, page 369) which will not reach adult size until the age of ten or eleven. Bacteria, which love hiding in these small crevices, can be difficult to dislodge and so at this age your child may have an almost constantly runny nose.

By the age of two, the pelvic bones have grown and spread to allow the abdominal contents to drop down into this area. Also at this age, the neck becomes more pronounced as the shoulder girdle and upper chest also descend. The ribs, too, start to shift position. Until now, they have lain horizontally, which is why small children find it difficult to breathe thoracically and, instead, persist in using the diaphragm to raise and lower the chest cavity.

Schoolkid Skeletons

In healthy kids, the rate of bone growth is faster than the rate of bone loss, so up to the teens and beyond, bones are still growing and strengthening. (Between thirty and forty – Mum and Dad's age – bone growth and bone loss are balanced. After fifty, poor granny's age, bone regeneration slows down and bone loss increases, giving rise to an overall deficit, but that's another book!)

By school age the sinuses are growing, which should mean fewer infections and fewer runny noses now. The height of your child will be a reflection of his or her genetic inheritance – birth weight and parents' height – but social and environmental factors can play a role too. Studies show that a significant proportion of the children born to families who have suffered long-term unemployment, for example, fail to reach their predicted growth targets by school entry.

One good thing about the list of foods that are helpful in maintaining strong bones in school-age kids is that it includes that childhood staple baked beans, which is a brilliant source of the ipriflavone the body needs to utilize all the other bone-building nutrients. (For an even healthier and more authentic alternative to the commercial varieties see Boston Baked Beans, page 219.) Dried fruits, such as apricots, prunes and dates, are another good source of bone-strengthening nutrients, so pack these into lunchboxes on schooldays.

Save soft fizzy drinks for an occasional treat. They contain phosphoric acid, which strips calcium from the bones. In one trial, for example, researchers found that children drinking six glasses of soft carbonated drinks per day had lower levels of calcium than other kids.

One of the growth hormones that targets skeletal muscles and bones is called somatotropin. This is a protein that causes cells to grow and then divide. In childhood, levels of growth hormone will rise eight or nine times a day, staying raised for between ten and twenty minutes. Usually these 'growth bursts' take place at night.

Teen Bones and Teeth

This is the time when your child becomes all fingers and toes, and there's a good anatomical reason for that – in adolescence, the feet and hands grow first, then the calves and forearms, the hips and chest, and finally the shoulders. Clumsiness at this time can simply be a sign that the brain has not yet recognized these growth spurts and the spatial changes they have brought to the body.

This is also when the jaw drops and the sex hormones kick in. Teen boys get stronger-looking shoulders and narrower hips, while girls develop wider and shallower pelvises and start to lay down fat deposits. This can then, with girls, set up an unhealthy cycle of crash dieting, which will have a knock-on effect on bone strength.

Sticks and Stones and Soft Drinks and Smoking

You may have laid the foundations for strong and healthy bones and teeth in your child's young life but if you have a teen daughter who has been yo-yo dieting or even a child who's hooked on soft, fizzy drinks, they may be undoing all your good work. And even if you've switched your family to healthy breakfast cereals and tried to do your best, you may have unwittingly robbed their bones of calcium by becoming one of what orthopaedic nurses and doctors – who anecdotally are reporting increasing numbers of minor fractures in teen girls – scathingly call 'those semi-skimmed Muesli Mums'.

The body needs calcium for blood clotting and for transmitting signals in the nerve cells, as well as for building bones, but it is one of the two most common deficiencies in menstruating females. (The other is iron.) And this deficiency is always worse in those who (a) eat junk diets which fail to provide enough calcium and bone-supporting micronutrients in the first place and

(b) those who have a history of yo-yo dieting.

What happens when the body does not get enough calcium in the diet is that it simply steals it from the bones, leaving them weakened and at risk of a fracture in later life. You may think this is irrelevant to your teen, but today there are over 3 million adult osteoporosis sufferers in the UK and more women now die from this condition than from cancer of the ovaries, cervix and uterus combined.

If you care about your daughter's health, you need to take steps now to reinforce the presence in the diet of calcium, ipriflavone and all the other micronutrients described here, throughout her childhood and puberty. If you plan to give her a supplement, remember that giving calcium on its own is not enough.

Smoking also destroys strong bones and the numbers of teenage girls smoking have long outstripped the numbers of boys. (Most start smoking to show off and then carry on to control their weight.) Coffee too increases the loss of calcium from the body, and so does salt in the diet, so try to limit the consumption of both by your teenagers.

Oxalic acid, a substance found in chocolate and rhubarb, can prevent the full absorption of any calcium they do eat, and too much fat in the diet will have the same effect. Rhubarb is easy to leave out but cutting back on the chocolate is going to require more monitoring by Mum and Dad.

Building good bone mass for the future throughout childhood is crucial – the more they start with, the more they can afford to lose – and if there is no underlying dairy allergy, then reintroducing full-fat milk will go a long way to help. In one study of teen girls who were given a pint of milk a day to drink for eighteen months, researchers recorded that average bone density increased by 3 per cent. And luckily for these researchers (and all the mums who supported the trial), the girls' weight stayed exactly the same. If you don't want to use milk, see page 174 for alternatives to dairy products. Remember, 90 per cent of bone mass has been laid down by adolescence in both sexes.

*****

Five-star Tip

Exercise is crucial for building a strong skeleton but it needs to be the right kind. Football and skipping will both build strong bones, so will walking, but swimming, which is not weight-bearing, won't. Preschoolers need at least an hour of free play a day. Encourage climbing, walking, riding bikes and kicking balls, all of which will help mould a strong skeleton.

The Fluoride Debate

Fluoride is a cumulative poison and has been banned in most of Europe and yet despite the results of worldwide trials showing no significant difference in tooth decay between children living in fluoridated and non-fluoridated communities, more than 90 per cent of us here still use fluoride toothpaste believing it will strengthen teeth and prevent cavities.

Since 1990, numerous large-scale studies have reported a link between fluoride intake and hip fractures in later life, and skeletal fluorosis is now said to be a serious risk in people who have ingested 10–20mg of fluoride per day for between ten and twenty years. The question is, how would you know how much you'd swallowed?

You can minimize this risk to your family by switching to organic, fluoride-free toothpastes. For kids, the Green People Company, which is dedicated to a chemical-free lifestyle for all, makes a mandarin flavour, and the toothpaste has no sodium lauryl sulphate – which is used in conventional products as a foaming agent but can dissolve protein in the body and so make gums weaker.

• To mail-order **Green People Company** products call 01444 401444.

Gut Feelings

What is digestion? It's that process where food is broken down into simple molecules that can then be absorbed by the blood or lymphatic system to be transported around or flushed out of the body. Naturopaths – natural healers who treat sickness without resorting to prescription medicines and who rely instead on homeopathy, nutrition and herbalism – reckon that even when everything works, it takes some 80 per cent of the body's total energy to complete this task. They also argue that digestive disorders – when things have gone wrong – are at the root of most chronic health problems. In other words, whatever the sickness you are dealing with, don't ignore what's going on with the digestion.

Children need all the same nutrients as adults, and health experts work out the recommended daily allowance (RDA) for children over the age of seven based on body weight (see Supplements, page 64). Most supplements, unless it says otherwise, are not suited to children under the age of three because before that age the digestive tract is not yet fully formed and so the gut is more permeable than in an older child.

The lining of the mature gut is naturally perforated with tiny sieve-like holes which allow essential nutrients to pass through into the bloodstream but keep larger molecules, which could cause problems, out. Many toddlers are prone to food intolerances (see page 169) and may react badly to, say, milk, which is high in a protein called casein, a larger molecule that has been shown to trigger an allergic-type reaction which can then cause eczema on the skin.

The syrups and powders that have been formulated for infants and children under the age of three are safe to use as recommended but always check the label to rule out artificial sweeteners and to work out the correct dosages.

Also key to good health in childhood and beyond is a healthy balance between the good bacteria in the gut, which work to help with digestion and which produce substances that boost the immune system and beat off stress, and those harmful bacteria that live alongside them. When this balance becomes out of kilter, the whole body will suffer. Thankfully, keeping the balance right can be as simple as giving your child a good quality probiotic supplement (see page 95), which is made up of replacement good bacteria.

If you have a baby with colic, use natural remedies, including a probiotic, to support the gut. If you have a schoolchild who is lactose intolerant, adopt the same treatment plan (see page 349). If you have a teen whose life is being ruined by acne, again go back to the gut and rebuild levels of the so-called 'friendly' bacteria (see page 289). In other words, optimum health always starts from the inside out and one of the most important places to start is the digestive system, which runs, of course, from the mouth to the anus.

Babies

When a baby is born, it is suddenly separated from the nutrients it was getting from the mother's blood via the placenta, and this shock can cause a dramatic 5–10 per cent drop in body weight. All babies are born with the senses of taste and smell, and since breastmilk is sweet, most breastfed babies are quite happy to take fresh fruits as their first solid foods. The ability to suck, bite, chew and swallow semi-solid food develops at around five months and by six or seven months your child will be able to tolerate 'lumpy' foods. That said, many children continue to gag or spit out lumps for many more months.

As your baby feeds, it takes in gas as well as milk. A 3.5kg baby will take in 100ml of milk during a 15-minute feeding session – and the same volume of air. The best position to hold a baby in to 'burp' them and help relieve discomfort from the gas is the sitting position with the back and neck supported. This allows the gas to rise back up a straightened windpipe or oesophagus.

A newborn has a stomach capacity of 10–20ml (a figure that will increase to 210–360ml by the child's first birthday) and will take two to three hours to empty its stomach. Although at birth there is not enough hydrochloric acid in the stomach to facilitate the digestion of protein, within the first eight hours of life the gastric juices begin to flow.

In infancy, the stomach plays an important role in coagulating curd or casein – the protein in milk – and controlling its passage into the large intestine. Although the whey in milk will move through the stomach within an hour, the curd can stay in the stomach for as long as twenty-four hours, slowly being broken down. In some babies, it is the digestion of the milk protein casein that is the root cause of problems, including colic (for natural remedies to treat this, see page 313). In the first six months of life, the body also produces very little pancreatic amylase – an enzyme which is used to digest complex carbohydrates – and this too has been highlighted as an underlying cause of colic. Researchers at the Department of Experimental Research at the University of Lund in Sweden report that 25 per cent of all babies with mild to moderate colic are indeed reacting to cow's milk. They pinpointed several signs of abnormal intestine function in colicky infants and recommended that breastfeeding mothers **adopt a strict dairy-free diet** and take calcium supplements. Formula-fed infants should also be taken off cow's milk and given a hypoallergenic, casein-hydrolysate formula instead.

Toddlers

Most children under the age of one have a problem digesting cow's milk and when toddlers are given milk as their main food, they are also at risk of developing an iron-deficiency anaemia (see Supplements, page 84). From six months, a variety of food is needed to provide all the vitamins, minerals and other nutrients a growing child needs. Vitamin C, for instance, cannot be stored by the body and so must be replaced every day (see Supplements, page 73) and parents who fall for marketing hype proclaiming a packet of crisps to contain more vitamin C than an apple need to remember we don't eat apples for their vitamin C content (which is low) but for their fibre and anti-inflammatory quercetin. One of the richest natural sources of vitamin C is not oranges but kiwi fruits (see a delicious recipe for kiwi salsa on page 224). If you do plan to give your child a vitamin C supplement, use one combined with a bioflavonoid such as quercetin, bilberry or rosehip, which will enhance its action in the body. (See Synergy, page 176.) I like **Biocare's Children's Vitamin C and Bilberry**. Mail-order on 0121 433 3727.

Another common digestive disorder in toddlers and younger schoolkids is an inability to digest milk sugar. This is not the same as a milk allergy (where the milk can be digested but still causes problems with the immune system) but is due to a lack of or deficiency in the enzyme **lactase,** which is manufactured in the small intestine where it splits the milk sugar lactose into glucose and galactose. **Nutrition Now's Lacto Safe** is formulated specifically for kids to aid this process. Its costs £6.95 for 45 tablets and is safe for children aged two and upwards. Mail-order on 0800 413596.

Toddlers devote around seven per cent of the energy they derive from food to growth (as opposed to maintenance and repair of the body tissues and activity), which is why old-fashioned nannies would serve calorie-packed nursery foods. Snacking is frowned on but since it is clearly here to stay (see page 165), serve healthier snacks and save crisps and more processed foods for an occasional treat. Preschool children (aged 1–5) do not in fact need as many calories as infants. What small children need to support their digestive system and growth are smaller, more frequent and varied meals.

Most toddlers have fairly regular bowel movements – potty training is always easier when you know your child will probably 'poo' after a meal – but until the age of two, this is more of a reflex action than any sign of toilet control. Small children do not have the developed nervous system that is needed to effect bowel control. All that happens is that a stool is passed once the rectum is full.

Schoolkids

Although most children have developed bowel control by the time they start school, this can be such a traumatic change that temporary regression is not uncommon. Your child may feel shy about sharing toilets with strangers for the first time or may not know how to ask to be excused. If this is a concern in your family, rest assured it will pass. Consistent soiling in children over four is, however, not normal and will need investigating.

In school-age kids, the emptying time for the stomach increases to between three and six hours; the stomach capacity increases to between 750 and 900ml by the age of ten. By this age acid levels in the stomach have risen so that in most children protein digestion is no longer a problem. However, most families in the West eat more than enough protein, and a greater concern is the limited amount of fruit and vegetables our kids are eating. Between the ages of four and ten, the daily protein requirement per kilogram of body weight drops from 1.5g to 1.2g per kg per day. Your child may also have an underlying food intolerance or allergy linked to animal proteins from milk and dairy products that is causing digestive upset and which you will need to tackle (see Food Intolerances, page 169).

The key supplement to give schoolchildren to support the digestive system is a probiotic or, even cleverer, a combined pre- and probiotic. Again, I rate one of the supplements from the US digestive-disorder specialist Nutrition Now. **Rhino FOS and Acidophilus** tastes of raspberry and comes in a kid-friendly bottle of sixty chewable tablets. Only available from Victoria Health, and safe for children aged one and upwards, you can mail-order this supplement on 0800 413596.

Teens

Ask a teen to keep a food diary and you'll find they get most of their nutrients from bread, chips, milk (unless they're dieting), biscuits, meat, cakes and pudding. Most parents of kids in their mid-teens have little control over what their offspring are eating – and what they're eating is the high-fat, high-sugar, low-fibre diet that has been implicated, time and time again, in the nation's two biggest killers in adulthood: cancer and heart disease.

By sixteen, the stomach capacity has increased to 1,500ml, which is still a lot smaller than the 2,000–3,000ml average adult capacity. Yet what self-respecting teen is going to walk into McDonald's or any other fast-food restaurant and ask for a kid's Happy Meal or children's size portion? They won't. They'll expect, get and eat as much, if nor more, than you. (See Obesity, page 14.)

Food diaries of teenagers reveal how the majority eat almost no fruits or vegetables and drink little or no pure water. The upshot? They may be trendy Generation X but the chances are that most of them are secretly and severely constipated (see page 314) too. **Biocare's Children's Digestaid** provides all the enzymes that help the body break down fats, carbohydrates and proteins – however good or bad the diet. It includes amylase which digests carbohydrates, lipase which digests fats and oils, and bromelain and papain which both work to digest protein. Available in veggie capsules (if your child can't swallow them then break open the capsule to release the contents into food or juice), you can mail-order direct from the manufacturer on 0121 433 3727. Poor digestion may be a result of a hidden food intolerance, a poor diet or other digestive disorder. Whatever the reason, this supplement, especially when taken with a good quality probiotic (see page 95), will help restore optimum health.

*****

Five-star Tip

Not something to talk about over breakfast but if you have a case of threadworm in the family – and 40 per cent of kids under ten are infected, however clean your home – then you need to adopt a regimen to first kill off the parasite, then expel it, and finally prevent re-infection. For kids, use grapefruit seed extract which is now widely on sale and which has fantastic antiparasitic properties. Use as directed on the bottle and disguise in a non-acidic fruit juice such as apple. Also cut back on sugar in the diet until the treatment ends. To prevent re-infection, use a tincture of black walnut and wormwood made by Nature's Answer and on sale in most good health stores.

Lung Power

The figures for childhood asthma have doubled in the last fifteen years – in some regions, as many as one in four children will now be asthmatic – and while we now know much more about the mechanism of asthma, nobody seems any closer to a cure. Understanding how the lungs develop through childhood and how you can use nutrition and herbs to support these changes can help minimize the risk of a lifetime dependency on inhalers and steroids for your child. For specific advice on coping with asthma and other respiratory problems, including chest infections and bronchitis, see the A–Z Guide, page 305. Here, we will look at general support you can give to the developing lungs and airways, which don't even reach maturity until the age of eight.

The anti-inflammatory properties of the fish oils rich in **omega-3** and **omega-6** fatty acids can help keep airways clear, especially when the underlying cause of infection is an allergic reaction. When choosing a brand, avoid heavy metal contamination and other ocean pollutants by making sure you buy a marine fish oil that is as pure as you can get. **Higher Nature's** fish oil capsules come from an unpolluted source. Ninety 500mg capsules cost £4.70. Call 01435 882880 for mail order. Give two a day.

Natural remedies which work in the body to support the lungs and airways include vitamins C and B12. Vitamin C is wiped out by cigarette smoking, so if you know your teen is puffing away, and you plan to get them to take a supplement, make sure you add another 35mg a day to the age-appropriate dosage (see Supplements, page 73).

Herbs can be useful in supporting the airways too. Lobelia extract, for example, works in the body to relax the smooth muscles of the bronchial airways. Keep a bottle of **Lobelia Cough Syrup** from Napiers (0131 343 6683; 100ml costs £4.25) in the cupboard for chesty coughs and emergencies but don't give this herb internally for more than a week or two.

In Australia, where asthma rates are even higher than here, a natural remedy called **Oralmat** which contains **rye grass** is used to help support lung function in asthma and other respiratory problems. Rye grass contains calming **tryptophan**, one of the chemicals the brain needs to make the feel-good mood-booster serotonin, plus **zinc** which strengthens the immune system too. It also contains magnesium, which helps keep both muscles and immune function healthy. In trials at the John Hunter Hospital in Newcastle, Australia, forty adult patients were given an extract of rye grass or a placebo for four weeks. Researchers found those taking the rye grass not only felt better but could exercise for longer and had better lung function after just one week.

Dr Chris Reynolds was the first medical doctor in Australia to use Oralmat in his clinic. In an article published in the journal of the Australian Naturopathic Practitioners and Chiropractors' Association, he admits he too was surprised by how effective it was: 'It is inexpensive, not unpleasant to take and easy to administer,' he reports. 'I believe it could replace many traditional drugs, eliminate the unwanted side effects and help treat many respiratory illnesses.' Oralmat, which is also reported to be effective against other allergies, plus colds, flu, respiratory problems, viral, fungal and bacterial infections, is now on sale in health stores here. It costs around £28 for 10ml. Mail-order from the **Nutri Centre** on 020 7436 5122. To give it, place two drops under the tongue and tell your child to let it stay there for fifteen seconds before swallowing. Repeat three times a day.

Baby Breath

On day twenty-six of a new pregnancy, two tiny buds begin to branch out from the trachea – buds that over the next twelve weeks will develop into your baby's lungs. From twenty-four weeks to birth, the air sacs (where the exchange of oxygen and carbon dioxide into and out of the blood takes place) develop, and by the time your baby is born, each lung will have up to 70 million of these tiny but crucial air sacs or alveoli. (In an adult, the number is closer to 400 million.)

In the womb, the lungs are filled with fluid and only about 8 per cent of the total blood volume will circulate to this area – just enough to keep the pulmonary tissues nourished. By the second half of a pregnancy, the baby will show frequent, shallow and irregular breathing movements, and one of the most important things a newborn will do in the first seven days of life is to switch from this irregular, often ineffectual pattern of breathing to a regular and rhythmic system that signals the full adaptation to air breathing.

Many babies alternate periods of rapid breathing with periods of a slower rate of breath. They may not breathe at all for periods of up to fifteen seconds, which is perfectly normal, as long as their colour and heart rate don't change too dramatically. This is known as apnoea, and is common in babies under thirty-two weeks. To trigger spontaneous breathing again, gently flick the bottom of one of the feet with your fingers. If you are at all worried, call the doctor.

Toddler Breath

From birth until the age of three, the number of immature alveoli (air sacs) is increasing. After three, it is the size, not the number, of these structures that increases. As new air sacs form, so do the new blood vessels that service them. At this age, the ribs lie horizontally and so most of the effort to move the ribcage for breathing comes from the diaphragm – a dome-shaped muscle that lies under the ribs and over the stomach. The anatomy books tell us this is a very inefficient way to breathe, yet it is the way we relearn to breathe when we adopt the pranayama (breathing techniques) of ha tha yoga, and is the way most musicians and singers breathe.

Heat and water are transmitted from the body's tissues to the air we breathe in and out. In small children, this loss is relatively high. The loss of water is also the reason younger children are more likely to suffer from a build-up of thicker mucus or mucus 'plugs' in the airways when in the throes of a respiratory infection.

Schoolkid Breath

Even at the age of five, the respiratory system and its airways are not fully formed. The air sacs, where carbon dioxide waste is exchanged for a fresh supply of oxygen, are still forming and so oxygen is not being delivered to the body tissues as economically as it could be. To compensate, and especially during activity, which in kids this age tends to be in short, fast bursts, your child will breathe more quickly and more shallowly – in effect, hyperventilate – which will help to oxygenate the blood more quickly.

The fact is that children's oxygen uptake is at least as good as an adult's but their body movements are less efficient. Another reason that breathing is more of an effort at this age is that the intercostal muscles between the ribs are still weak and hold only limited stores of glycogen, which the body burns to make energy. This in turn will restrict respiratory capacity, limiting not only how much exercise a child this age can do but how long they can keep it up.

The air sacs continue to develop until the age of eight, by which time the respiratory system is so sophisticated that as well as the airways, tubes and sacs it needs to allow the body to breathe, it will have also developed specialized pathways to allow trapped gas in obstructed airways to become reabsorbed into the body.

> *****
> *Five-star Tip*
> Between the age of five and puberty, the weight of the lungs will increase three-fold, and so for mums coping with kids who suffer from asthma it is important to check that the inhalers and equipment they are using are appropriate to their age and development.

Teenage Lungs

Gender differences in the respiratory systems begin to show shortly before puberty when, thanks to a surge of testosterone, boys develop greater muscle mass and a higher haemoglobin concentration (haemoglobin is the substance in the red blood cells that transports oxygen around the body) than girls of the same age.

From the age of eight to sixteen, the maximum uptake of oxygen for boys increases by 150 per cent. For the same period with girls, the increase is just 80 per cent. For girls – and they won't thank you for mentioning this – it is the pre- and post-pubescent accumulation of body fat that makes the difference. Lean muscle has a higher metabolic rate and thus demands more oxygenated blood than fat.

Researchers tell us that eating lots of antioxidant-rich fruits and vegetables (see Food Talk, pages 157–232) can help protect the lungs in childhood and beyond, yet study after study shows that kids in affluent societies are eating almost *no* fruits and vege-tables, never mind the recommended five portions a day. (This is five combined portions, not five of each, though for optimum health the true figure is closer to eight portions.) Food diaries of teenagers show how it is not untypical for a seven-day diary covering twenty-one meals to include almost no vegetables, fruits or water, and this is not that much worse than the findings among the under-fives. Mind you, are we grown-ups any better? Not according to US nutritionist and author Carol Simonatacchi who warns, 'Adults don't eat any better than kids, according to national statistics and my own client records. The level of nutrition in the Western culture, upper or lower class, is appalling.'

The Heart of the Matter

When children as young as ten have been diagnosed with the early signs of atherosclerosis or furring of the arteries, you know the next generation is in trouble. The American Heart Association has already warned parents to watch the saturated fat intake of children as young as two, and, just as shocking, millions of kids aged six to seventeen are being diagnosed as suffering from high blood pressure.

In reality, the moment a child is born, the arterial blood vessels start to fur. According to clinical studies, children as young as one have fatty streaks in their blood vessels, and 26 per cent of all kids aged two to twelve have raised cholesterol levels. This does not mean your child will have heart problems now but it can mean problems in later life unless you introduce healthier habits and lifestyle choices early on. There is no quick-fix natural supplement that is going to keep your child's heart and blood vessels healthy for life. Instead, you are going to have to use diet and lifestyle to swing the odds back in favour of a longer life and away from a high risk of heart disease in adulthood.

Keeping cholesterol levels under control has become accepted as one way of reducing the risk of heart disease in adults, but the body needs cholesterol to make vitamin D (which is actually a hormone) from sunlight, to make the sex hormones from puberty onwards and to make the fatty sheaths that cover nerve fibres. In fact, most of the cholesterol in the body is made by the liver. What is of more significance in adults – and because of the ethics of running clinical trials using minors as guinea pigs nobody has yet asked or investigated if this applies to kids – are levels of another substance in the blood called **homocysteine**. This is an amino acid and a natural by-product of normal metabolism which is now thought to promote plaque formation in adults and which is said to be forty times more accurate as a predictor for heart problems than cholesterol levels.

Raised homocysteine levels have been found in the blood of 40 per cent of adult patients suffering from heart disease and there is a growing body of evidence linking high levels of this substance with an increased risk of heart problems, independent from other risk factors including high cholesterol or high blood pressure. (Around 80 per cent of all fatal heart attacks, for example, occur in men who do not have high cholesterol levels.) Smoking cigarettes and drinking lots of coffee are both now linked with higher risks of heart disease in adults – what is less well known is that they have been associated with higher levels of homocysteine too.

A healthy body detoxifies homocysteine by converting it back to methionine, the substance from which it was produced in the first place, or by breaking it down even further to form a more harmless substance called cystathionine. Things that can interfere with this process include either a genetic fault in one of the enzymes responsible for this chemical breakdown or a deficiency in any one of the nutrients needed to activate these enzymes in the first place.

The most important nutrients for regulating the breakdown of homocysteine are **vitamins B6, B12** and **folic acid**. For kids over twelve, you can safely buy adult supplements and give an age-related dosage (see Supplements, page 65). And since all the B vitamins work best when taken together (see Synergy, page 88), the best supplement to give is a good **B complex**. Healthwise mums and dads will also try to increase foods that are rich in these nutrients in the family diet. For the B vitamins these include wheatgerm and brewer's yeast – which can both be hidden in smoothies (see page 195) – cabbage, eggs, cantaloupe melons, cheese and red meats (use lean cuts to reduce saturated-fat intake) and, for folic acid, dark green leafy vegetables, beans, wholewheat and rye breads, carrots, pumpkins and apricots.

Stressed-out Kids

Risk factors for coronary heart disease in later life include smoking, a junk diet, obesity (see page 14) and taking no exercise. Sound like any kids you know? Add a daily dose of childhood stress, emotional upsets following family breakdowns and divorce, and you can see how this gameboy generation of couch potato kids may not live long enough to watch their own grand-children and great-grandchildren discover sex 'n' drugs and rock 'n' roll.

The two key **antistress nutrients** are **co-enzyme Q10** (CoQ10) and **carnitine** – both of which shot to fame in gyms where they were being used by body builders to enhance strength, stamina and endurance. CoQ10 is found in every single cell in the body and plays a key role in energy production. Carnitine is produced naturally in those organs that work the hardest – the brain, heart and kidneys. It is used to transport fatty acids into the mito-chondria (power stations) of the cells to be converted into energy for the heart and skeletal muscles. Both nutrients are now sold in health stores in supplement form for adults and you can give an adult dosage to teens aged fifteen and over. For younger kids, you will have to be clever about the food choices you make and incorporate more of both nutrients into the family diet.

According to studies published in the *American Journal of Cardiology*, adult heart patients taking co-enzyme Q10 (which can also help lower blood pressure) lived three years longer than a control group that was not given this supplement. Foods that are rich in **CoQ10** include **spinach, tuna, sardines, beef** (which is also a good source of carnitine) and, if there is no underlying allergy, **peanuts. Red meat** and **dairy products** are the best food sources of **carnitine** but parents then face a Catch 22 since these are the very foods that are also high in plaque-promoting saturated fats. The solution? Use lean cuts and for older kids (fifteen-plus) use a carnitine supplement. To beat stress, give all kids a good **B-complex** supplement.

The herbal remedy **Hawthorn Berry Extract** which is widely on sale and more traditionally used to treat bad breath in kids also has heart-protecting benefits. Use a tincture and give at-risk children over twelve an age-appropriate dose (see Phytomedicine, page 101).

Essential fatty acids (EFAs) help reduce cholesterol throughout childhood and will provide some protection against heart disease in later life. **Essential Balance Jnr** from Omega Nutrition is organic and provides a 1:1 ratio of omega-3 and omega-6 fatty acids. Mail-order from the Nutri Centre (020 7436 5122).

The Newborn Heart

At birth, the heart occupies 40 per cent of the space of what is called the lung field – a figure that drops to 30 per cent in adulthood. In other words, the newborn has a bigger heart, proportionally, than its mother. For the first eight weeks of life, the demand for oxygen is high and anything that increases that demand, say a cold or sepsis (which is a bacterial infection of the bloodstream), will also stress the heart. The average pulse of a newborn is 145 beats per minute, which drops to 115 beats per minute by the first birthday.

The Schoolkid's Heart

Children's hearts pump a smaller volume of blood and have to beat faster to oxygenate their tissues but from the age of three to fifteen the ratio of heart mass to body mass slowly declines.

What a child eats, and levels of anxiety and excitement, can all change the heart rate and so although the average pulse for a five-year-old is 95 beats per minute, this can increase up to a maximum of 200 beats per minute, depending on what the child is doing.

At the age of six gender differences take hold, with females having higher heart rates than males. Boys also then start to show faster recovery rates after exercise than girls and other cardio-vascular changes that give them the edge when it comes to endurance sports. The resting blood pressure rises throughout childhood as the heart grows bigger and stronger.

Overweight children have a higher pulse rate because their heart has to pump harder to circulate blood around the adipose (fat) tissue that has been stored. But underweight kids may have a higher pulse rate too. The theory here is that these kids may be more anxious and have more adrenaline pumping, which also works to speed up the heart rate.

By fifteen, the average pulse is seventy beats per minute; less than half that of the newborn child. By the early teens, most youngsters will also have some evidence of atheroma or plaque deposits. What researchers don't know is whether these are permanent or reversible, and whether they will only be a problem if the wrong lifestyle choices are made. What we do know is that a diet that is low in animal fats and junk foods will reduce blood cholesterol levels in all age groups, including teens.

Fighting Force – The Immune System

The most important thing to know about the immune system is that scientists are still a long way from understanding how it all works. Immunology is still a relatively new field of study. Even newer is psychoneuroimmunology, which recognizes that how someone feels and what is going on in their life will have a direct effect on their immune response. In other words, when it comes to the body's natural defences, you cannot treat the body alone and simply ignore the mind.

A child's immune system is not fully developed before the age of fourteen, making kids under this age particularly susceptible to infection and sickness. What little immunity they do start life with is passed on from the mother via the placenta (before birth) and then in breastmilk. This is known as passive immunity and is fairly short-lived. A more active and longer-lasting immunity is acquired following exposure to infection which then stimulates the immune system to respond. This exposure can be to an infection like chicken pox, caught from another child, or through immunization (see pages 5–13).

The role of the immune system is to protect the body from invaders, whether it's a microbe, a cancer cell or a transplant organ. Its workings are complex, involving different organs, specialized cells, hormone messengers and the intricate lymphatic system which permeates every organ in the body except the brain. The immune system may be complicated but its mission is always simple – to recognize the enemy, mobilize forces and attack. The enemy? Teeming hordes of micro-organisms (bacteria, viruses, parasites and fungi) which want to move in for free food and shelter, and our own cells when they mutate and become cancerous.

So a key player in keeping the body healthy is the lymphatic system. The lymphatic vessels contain lymph (a pale, thick fluid made up of a fatty liquid and white blood cells) and built into this network are special areas, including the lungs, intestines, bone marrow, spleen, liver, tonsils and lymph nodes, where the infection-fighting lymphocyte cells can be recruited, mobilized and dispatched to where they are needed. The reason lymph nodes swell is that the infection is drained from, say, an open wound to these and other sites where the lymphocytes can then destroy and clear it.

The body's first defence against infection and disease actually has nothing to do with the immune system but rests with the skin and the protective mucosal surfaces. This is thanks to the presence of an antimicrobial enzyme called lysozyme which will break down the cell walls of invading organisms. Lysozyme is present throughout our lives in body sweat, in tears and in saliva. The acidity of the digestive juices also helps to protect the body from infection and the presence of beneficial microflora in the gut, mouth, upper respiratory tract and skin provides an additional protective barrier. However, when infection does penetrate these barriers, the immune system kicks in.

The immune response is always activated by the lymphocytes – special mobile cells found in the blood, thymus gland, lymph nodes, spleen and tissue spaces. There are two types of lymphocytes, known as B cells and T cells, each with a different way of defending the body. The T cells will have a head-on, direct fight with an invading organism (antigen), while the B cells will produce special chemicals called antibodies (immunoglobulins) to destroy the antigen.

What's clever about the lymphocytes is that they can (a) tell the difference between the body's own tissue and the antigen, (b) produce specific antibodies to destroy specific antigens and (c), even more extraordinary, hold a 'memory' of previous invasions and recognize antigens they have destroyed before. Lymphocytes are also self-regulating and are programmed to deactivate themselves once the antigen (the infection) has been cleared from the body.

Supporting Children's Immune Systems

For kids of all ages the immune system's biggest enemy is stress and it's important to remember that events which would not faze an adult may be highly stressful to a child. Obvious stressors include moving to a new school, coping with parents' divorce, sitting exams, the arrival of a new child in the family, and the conflicting emotions surrounding puberty, bullying and peer pressure. A weakened immune system is all too often the underlying cause of many everyday childhood health problems, and even when there are no obvious signs of sickness, supporting the immune system through stressful events – and even seasonal changes – will pay dividends in terms of your child's health both now and in the longer term.

If stress, pollution and poor diet are the immune system's enemies then its best friends are good nutrition, R&R (antistress chill-out time with rest and relaxation) and good antioxidant support to clear out the free radicals that are a normal by-product of metabolism but which can, if left unchecked, destroy tissues and weaken the immune response. (To learn more about anti-oxidants and free radicals, see page 182.)

There are four steps to take to support your child or children's immune system:

- Give them an immune-boosting herb.
- Give them a probiotic to replenish levels of the good gut bacteria that support the immune system.
- Give them a good multisupplement with all the antistress B vitamins.
- Give them a low-dose daily zinc supplement which helps 'tone' the immune system to keep it in peak condition.

The herbs

The best-known and best-selling of all the herbal immune boosters is **echinacea** (ek-in-a-shea). Suggestions that you can only use this herb for four to six weeks, after which time it loses its potency, have not been substantiated so a good tip is to give your kids a daily low dose for maintenance from 1 September to 30 March (the UK's autumn and winter) and only increase the dosage if they are showing signs of succumbing to sickness. **Nutrition Now's Rhino Echinacea** is made from *Echinacea purpurea* (don't waste your money on supplements made from other varieties) and is available in chewable tablets (£6.95 for 60) or in tincture form (£9.95 for 60ml). This range is only available from Victoria Health in the UK. Mail-order enquiries on 0800 413596.

Also, keep a bottle of **Elagen** in the bathroom cupboard for times when the immune system is low. The active ingredient is an

Asian plant called *Eleutherococcus senticosus*, which is related to immune-boosting and antistress ginseng and which is safe to give to children. Elagen costs £11.35 for 30 capsules and is available by mail order from a company called Eladon in Bangor, Wales (01248 370059).

The probiotic

A good probiotic will maintain healthy levels of the beneficial bacteria that also support the immune system. **Rhino FOS and Acidophilus,** from Nutrition Now (see above), provides a double whammy with not only replacement bacteria but also the food the bacteria need (FOS) to stay strong in the body, all in one powdered supplement.

The multisupplement

There are lots of good (and bad) multisupplements for kids. Check the label and rule out those which contain any of the artificial sweeteners, especially aspartame. If you want to stick to Nutrition Now's Rhino range, it includes the **Rhino Chewy Vites** for kids. I also like **Nature's Plus Animal Parade** which packs twenty-eight vitamins and minerals, including iron for healthy blood and choline for brain power, into the shape of lions, elephants, tigers and hippos. The shapes come in cherry, grape or orange flavour and are OK for vegetarians to take. Ninety animals cost £9.85. Mail-order from the Nutri Centre (020 7436 0422). **Solgar's Vita-Kid Multivitamin Wafers** are also excellent and free from starch and salt. For Solgar stockists call 01442 890355. For kids over twelve, you can use supplements formulated for adults and give an age-appropriate dosage.

The zinc

Back to the **Nutrition Now Rhino** range. Give an age-appropriate dose of this mineral which tones the immune system to help it function at optimum levels again. Each chewable tablet in this particular supplement provides 5mg of elemental zinc. The price is £5.95 for 60. Mail-order from Victoria Health on 0800 413596. For children over twelve, step up this dose to 12mg for girls and 15mg for boys.

Babies

The infant thymus gland, which plays a key role in organizing the immune response, is proportionately large and remains so throughout childhood. By week nine of a pregnancy, the first immune cells are starting to appear in the foetus's blood and tissues, and by week fifteen, some 65 per cent of the lymphocytes in the thymus gland are the destroyer T cells.

The immune system's antibody-producing B cells appear in the liver about a week after the T cells first appear. The B cells then migrate to the bone marrow, ready to produce the antibodies that will protect your baby at birth. The B cells secrete a number of different antibodies or immunoglobulins, which are then involved in different body systems. **IgA**, for instance, is concentrated in the respiratory and gastrointestinal tract (GI) and is found in saliva, tears and GI secretions. Scientists have found that breastfed babies are better protected from intestinal infections in early life, which suggests IgA is one of the immune factors passed on through breastmilk.

IgG is another important antibody which passes to the baby via the placenta. It identifies invading organisms and activates inflammation and the other blood and cell changes that respond to the presence of dead tissue, micro-organisms, toxins or any other foreign material. In pregnancy, this immunoglobulin is usually transferred during the third (final) trimester. (Premature babies may be deficient in this protective factor and are thus more at risk of infection.)

IgE is involved in allergic and the extreme anaphylactic reactions and has been found to be present in higher levels in children who suffer these types of reactions. **IgM** is another antibody which remains in the bloodstream where it reacts with foreign antigens in the blood. It accounts for around 10 per cent of all the antibodies present and is the main immunoglobulin produced in infancy.

Toddlers

A stressed-out toddler is not going to be able to tell you what's wrong but there are usually plenty of signs that your child is feeling overwhelmed, a state which, if not addressed, is going to batter the immune system. Typical signs of not coping include sudden incontinence, night terrors and aggressive or unusual behaviour with other children and adults.

Even before starting school your toddler is likely to have had five of the UK's recommended seven different vaccinations (see page 7 for how to support their immune system through these vaccines), so aside from everyday infections, their immune system will have now been exposed to at least seven very serious diseases, including polio and tetanus. Some babies are also given the tuberculosis (BCG) vaccination at birth, bringing this number to eight.

Schoolkids

School worries and repeated exposure to infections are all part of the everyday hazards children this age now face – all stressors which, again, will have an adverse effect on the immune system if not tackled. Signs of stress in a school-age child can include refusing to go to school, falling behind with homework and unexpectedly failing to meet normal reading and writing targets in school. Even if you can't wipe out the worries, you can take steps to give the immune system extra support during times of extra stress. Since the flower remedies support the system on a psychological and emotional level too, this would be a good time to give them to your child (see page 124). I like the Australian bush flower remedies and the two that support the thymus, which plays a key role in regulating immune response, are **Illawarra Flame Tree** and **Southern Cross**. These are safe for all ages.

Teens

Although doctors treat the internal systems of the human body as being 'adult' by the age of twelve, the immune system is not fully developed until the age of fourteen. Again, pressures that are particular to this age group, such as worrying about their changing body shape, peer pressure, exams, heightened sexuality and confrontational run-ins with the parents, can all cause an accumulation of stress which will then have a negative knock-on effect on the immune system. Recurrent infections are a sign of immune stress in all age groups. After fourteen, your child should not succumb to more than two colds a year: if teens are constantly catching colds or other infections, then you know their immune system is under stress and needs your help.

Talking Immunity

The only immune system jargon you'll ever need to know.

Antigen Any molecule capable of stimulating an immune response. Can be a bug, a virus, a toxin, a food or a splinter.

Antibody A protein made by the B lymphocyte cells that will react with a specific antigen. Also called an immunoglobulin.

Complement A group of proteins that helps attack antigens. Activated by IgM, one of the immunoglobulins that circulates in the blood.

Cytokines Soluble proteins secreted by the cells of the immune system which act as messengers to help regulate an immune response.

Immune response The response to an antigen by the components of the immune system, either cells or antibodies.

Interferon A protein released by cells to attack viruses (which cause colds, flu, mumps etc.) and stimulate Natural Killer Cells.

Lymphocytes The 'brains' of the immune system. Specialized **T cells** which can distinguish between self and non-self to find those invaders that hide inside the body's own cells; or **B cells** which produce antibodies to destroy antigens. These cells are also clever enough to remember previous antigens encountered – they can differentiate between up to a million different antigens – whether they entered the body through the lungs (breathing), the intestines (eating) or the skin (injury/surgery).

Macrophage A large cell that literally engulfs and ingests microbes after they have been targeted for destruction by the T cells.

Natural Killer Cells These do what their name says: they are a type of lymphocyte that can kill certain microbes and cancer cells. Invaded cells give themselves away by the abnormal proteins on their surface.

Hormone Havoc

Puberty lasts, on average, three years. It's not just one event, of course, but a whole series of changes to your child's body spread over those years and following a sequence that will be unique to each individual. One thing that varies enormously, for instance, is the age at which puberty starts. In boys it can be as young as ten or as old as sixteen, and in girls, although the age of onset can, again, vary widely, the average age in this country is now twelve.

The changes which signal your child is well on the way to adulthood (at least physically) are usually accompanied by a growth spurt and one of the less well-known triggers for puberty is the amount of body fat your child has accumulated. In girls, in the UK, a weight of around 47kg (roughly 7½ stone) has been suggested as the critical weight which triggers a change in both the metabolic rate and in the production of hormones. That said, this critical weight differs between cultures and nobody has yet published the comparable figure for boys.

During puberty and thanks to the influence of the female hormone oestrogen, girls not only acquire more body fat than boys, the fat they are carrying will be distributed differently, with females carrying more fat around the shoulders, hips and buttocks. At the end of puberty, your teen daughter will have up to 10 per cent more body fat than a male of the same age.

Babies

Girl babies are born with all the 400,000 eggs they will ever have. These are all present in the ovaries at birth, after which the number will start to decline. (Prescription drugs, injury and infection during childhood can all reduce the number of healthy ova.)

Babies of both sexes are often born with enlarged breasts. This is caused by the mother's hormones, which can also trigger a discharge of a clear fluid from the baby's breasts. Again, this is normal and will correct itself over the first few weeks of your child's life, so don't be alarmed.

In the last weeks of the last trimester of gestation of a male foetus, the testicles descend. At birth, the tubes that carry seminal fluid in males are solid and they remain that way until puberty when the testicles enlarge – adult testicles weigh forty times those of an infant – and these tubes become hollow.

Toddlers

Thanks to the influence of the male hormone, testosterone, your male children will already have a lower percentage of fat than your female children. This hormonal influence first starts to subtly manifest itself between the ages of three and four, and becomes increasingly marked throughout childhood towards puberty.

In all young children, the action of hormones is having an impact on their body shape. At this age, for instance, children have more fat over their arms and legs than on the trunk of their body. In puberty, boys lose this limb fat and accumulate fat on their trunk. In girls, as we have seen, the fat is laid down in more sex-specific areas such as the hips and breasts.

Schoolkids

Since birth the uterus in a girl has remained in the same position, but as the bladder starts to descend into the pelvic cavity (and this usually happens around the age of six) then the womb changes its position too. By the age of seven, it will have adopted the familiar tilted position of the adult womb. Throughout childhood, the ovarian tissue grows to a size that is twenty times its weight at birth.

When a male child is born, the prostate gland and the rectum are the only two organs found in the pelvic cavity. The prostate grows slowly throughout childhood, until puberty, when it suddenly doubles its size over a short period. After this the growth rate slows again until the adult prostate, which lies just under the bladder and which helps produce the seminal fluid that nourishes sperm, reaches the size of a small walnut, weighing in at around 25g, which is just 1oz.

Teens

In both sexes, the gland producing the hormone that acts on the testes and the ovaries is the pituitary, which is itself stimulated by hormones released by the hypothalamus gland. The pituitary gland produces two hormones, which have different actions in males and females. The first is **follicle stimulating hormone (FSH)** which, in females, stimulates the cycle that results in the maturation of one of the stored eggs. In males, it regulates the production of sperm in the testes.

The second of these two hormones is called **luteinizing hormone (LH)**. Again, it is produced in both sexes but has different actions in the sex organs. In girls, LH plays a role in the production of the two female hormones, oestrogen and progesterone. In boys, it stimulates the production of the male hormone, testosterone.

The other important hormones causing havoc in puberty are the **androgens**, produced from the adrenal glands which sit atop the kidneys. In both sexes, these stimulate the growth of hair under the arms and in the pubic areas, as well as bringing about changes in both the sweat and sebaceous skin glands. (In other words, it is these androgen hormones which cause the spots and smelly socks that teens and their mums worry and complain about.) The good news, of course, is that unless there is an underlying hormonal problem, both sexes can kiss goodbye to these more difficult aspects of puberty at the end of this rite of passage.

The Menstrual Cycle

For females, disruptions to the monthly menstrual flow and changes to the menstrual cycle can provide further clues to what is happening to the delicate hormonal balance that is being established.

The menstrual cycle, which can range from nineteen to thirty-six days (the average is twenty-eight days) is controlled by the hormones oestrogen and progesterone. Each month, the womb builds up a rich lining in preparation for the implantation of a fertilized egg. When this does not happen, levels of oestrogen (which promote this build-up) decline, and levels of progesterone (which trigger the shedding of the womb lining) rise instead.

To release the lining, the arteries go into spasm and release prostaglandins which play a role in killing off the cells of the lining. During a period around 50ml (three tablespoons) of blood, along with glandular secretions and tissue fragments from the inner wall of the womb, is shed. This blood does not clot until it reaches the vagina (the womb contains anticlotting enzymes) and the heavy clots that accompany a heavy flow are a combination of clumped red blood cells, mucus, glycogen and glycoproteins.

Painful periods are a common problem among teens. The reason for the pain is that the release of prostaglandins needed to help destroy and shed the lining of the womb can also trigger an inflammatory reaction in the womb which then responds with more muscle spasm. Even when there are no obvious problems, the menstrual cycle can change in response to emotional factors such as fear and stress, and even in response to smell. This is because the master hypothalamus gland, which controls the pituitary gland, which controls the sex hormones, is responding to all parts of the nervous system, which are themselves responding to the environment. In short, everything that is going on in your daughter's life will affect her hormone balance.

You can help the body to rebalance its hormones and to re-regulate its menstrual cycle by giving your teenage daughter **agnus castus**. This is an adaptogen – a herb that works to help the body perform better under everyday stress – and is used to regulate the pituitary gland which, as we have seen, controls the production of FSH and LH and, thus, the sex hormones. Numerous clinical trials carried out over the past thirty years show how agnus castus can help control the symptoms of PMT, including bloating, breast tenderness, backache, cramping, irritability and depression. It will also help get rid of associated teen and premenstrual acne. This herb is now so popular and so well known that it is widely on sale in all good health stores in both tincture and tablet forms.

- **For advice on specific hormonal problems such as Polycystic Ovary Syndrome (PCOS) and Endometriosis, see pages 363 and 332.**

The Good . . . Phytochemicals

What you can use to keep your children's hormones naturally balanced are foods that are rich in **phytoestrogens**. These are the plant chemicals that are not nutrients as such, but which confer a range of health benefits – including hormone balancing – when we eat them. Similar in structure to the female hormone oestrogen, they are only 1/1000th as potent and so when sourced from foods are completely safe for both sexes.

There are four main types of phytoestrogens (which are also known as isoflavones). These are:

- **genistein** (only found in soya)
- **daidzein** (found in soya, broccoli, garlic and peanuts)
- **formononetin** (found in red clover, chickpeas, lentils and mung beans)
- **biochanin** (also found in red clover, chickpeas, lentils and mung beans)

Phytoestrogens are present in over three hundred different plants, although the best food sources are soybeans, linseed (flaxseed), chickpeas and lentils. Other health-promoting phytochemicals found in foods include limonene from citrus fruits, dithiolthiones in Brussels sprouts, allium compounds found in garlic, and flavonoids found in most fresh fruits and vegetables.

The Bad . . . Xeno-oestrogens

Sperm count in the West has slumped by 50 per cent in the last five decades. One theory is that substances called xeno-oestrogens produced by chemicals used in the environment are responsible. You cannot rule out any exposure to these ecotoxins but you can take positive steps to minimize the risk and the harm. One step is to switch to organic food, where possible. The other is to store food in glass and not plastic containers. For example, keep left-overs in a glass bowl and stop using cling film. This would, of course, revolutionize the school lunchbox and, unfortunately, I've yet to track down a non-plastic substitute with Barbie on the front that would please my five-year-old!

The Ugly . . .

If you know or suspect your daughter is already having sex, talk to her about the importance of a barrier method of contraception and not just to prevent pregnancy. One of the most horrifying statistics I have discovered in my researches as a health writer is that within four years of becoming sexually active, 80 per cent of women (regardless of their age) are infected by the human papilloma virus (HPV), some strains of which can cause cervical cancer. Some 90 per cent of cervical carcinomas are believed to be related to an HPV infection – a deadly serious state of affairs. To learn more about how a natural health supplement can help protect your child from this risk, turn to page 112, which carries more information about coriolus, one of the Asian mushroom supplements which researchers believe may be able not only to control this virus but to reverse any damage already caused.

PART FIVE

An A–Z Guide to Natural Remedies for Everyday Complaints

Where to get them and how to use them

Introduction

In South America and other parts of the world, ordinary families have held on to the healing traditions that have been passed, usually from mother to daughter, from generation to generation. Native cultures know what to do and how to use the plants and foods that grow locally to help treat infection and ward off disease. But in the last century, ever since the NHS made health care free for all, we've lost almost all that traditional wisdom and put our faith, for the most part, in the healing powers of complete strangers. This is the section of the book that puts some of that knowledge back where it belongs . . . in your hands.

People are not 'born healers' and you don't have to be blessed by fairies or anything else New-Agey. The people who know how to use the information in this book have studied hard to resurrect much of it and there's no reason why you too can't become confident in safely using the same natural remedies in your home. When you do, you'll discover that children (like animals), who have no preconceived notions about what will or won't work, respond fantastically well to natural medicine, which, in turn, will boost your growing confidence.

The most important thing to remember is that the true definition of holistic – as in holistic health care – is that it treats the whole person and takes the best from all the systems available: conventional and alternative. So, for an acute condition, for an injury or a sickness that needs the high-tech skills of modern medicine, call the doctor. You can then use natural medicine to accelerate your child's recovery at home by, say, boosting the immune system or, after a course of antibiotics, rebalancing the flora in the digestive tract. For stubborn chronic conditions that can be managed but won't be cured by pills, look for the underlying cause and follow the suggestions in this section.

As a health journalist specializing in complementary medicine, I recognize there is a balance to be struck between scientific and empirical evidence. One lab experiment carried out on one mouse by one PhD doctorate student does not make any kind of a cure, however much the supplement manufacturers would like it to be so. And it would be arrogant to dismiss what we call empirical evidence, that is, if hundreds of thousands of people have taken a remedy and said it works, then they should be listened to. However, some of the remedies recommended here have undergone rigorous double-blind, placebo-controlled clinical trials (double-blind means neither tester nor subject knew who was getting what; placebo-controlled means the study included volunteers given nothing more than sugar pills), and you can't get better than that. In fact, one of the more rewarding aspects of working in this field is that, increasingly, mainstream researchers are able to identify the active ingredients in these traditional remedies and finally tell us how they really work.

In this A–Z guide to the very best of the natural remedies, you will find detailed information about the underlying causes of

288

everyday childhood and teenage complaints, plus up-to-date tips and advice for treating them. Whether it's eczema or nappy rash, acne or endometriosis, you will be told precisely what to use, how to use it and even where to get it. (We've included prices that were current at the time of going to press.)

If you don't have time to read more about what is going on, then simply scan the text for the key words, which we have highlighted in **bold**, so you know what you need to do and which herbs or supplements are going to help. Do take the time to check you are giving an age-related safe dosage (see our guidelines on pages 65, 101 and 120). You can then come back at your leisure, when the panic is over, to find out more about what is going on in your child's body. The next time you walk into a health store or call up their mail-order division, you'll know exactly what you need and why. Even better, you'll know from your own experience just how easy it is, once you start, to give your child the gift of long-lasting good health.

Acne

What's happening?

Contrary to popular belief, acne is not caused by junk diets or poor hygiene (although neither of these will help) but by a hormonal imbalance, the skin's reaction to this upset and a bacterium called *Propionibacterium acne* (*P. acne*) which has become increasingly resistant to the antibiotic creams and drugs that are the conventional treatment route.

The skin of acne sufferers has been found, for example, to exhibit greater activity of an enzyme called 5-alpha-reductase, which works to convert the male hormone, testosterone, to a more potent form called dihydrotestosterone. A **low-salt, calcium-rich diet** can help control an outbreak and so can one of the more calcium-rich but less well-known herbs, **red clover**. (Do not give supplements of red clover to teenage boys.)

Blood tests reveal higher levels of toxins from the gut flora of acne sufferers so give your teen a good quality **probiotic supplement** (see page 95) to counter this. In trials reported in the *British Journal of Dermatology*, researchers found daily **zinc supplements** (30mg a day) were as effective as oral antibiotics. **Vitamin B6** (50mg a day) can also help eliminate premenstrual flare-ups of acne and spots.

*****

Five-star Tip

If there is an acne or other skin outbreak, mix a little wheatgrass powder with warm water to make a paste, apply at night and leave it on the affected area until the morning.

What to take

Solgar's Red Clover veggie capsules cost £15.95 for 60. For stockists, call 01442 890355. **Xynergy's Sweet Wheat powder** costs £19.95 for 15g plus £1.95 p&p. To mail-order call 01730 813642. **Rio Trading** has an excellent anti-acne combination treatment which includes echinacea, red clover, burdock and chlorophyll: 30 veggie capsules cost £9.99. Use this company's **rosa mosqueta oil** (£9.99 for 20ml) for acne scars. Mail-order on 01273 570987. To keep skin clear of infection, use **Desert Essence face wash** with organic tea tree oil (£5.45 for 240ml).

Blackmore's Antibacterial Pimple Gel (£4.04 for 12ml) also contains tea tree, plus echinacea and antibacterial goldenseal.

Blackmore's one-a-day **Skin Support tablets** provide echinacea, zinc, calendula and betacarotene to help prevent and treat acne. 45 tablets cost £6.29. Mail-order from Revital (0800 252875).

I love the **Living Nature skincare** range which is 100 per cent natural. Formulated by a New Zealand-trained biochemist with a real feeling for herbs and a passion for manuka honey, the **acne kit** includes a purifying cleansing gel, a deep cleansing clay mask and peel, a manuka honey antiseptic gel, a balancing flax cream and a **Teen Skincare Guide** booklet. It costs £28.35. For more information, call 01489 566144.

The **Helen Sher skincare** system and make-up range is designed for both acne and rosacea skins. It is not cheap and will not work for everyone but is worth investigating for chronic conditions. For details, call 020 7499 4022. More affordable for most pockets, the **Botanical Therapeutic skincare** range is also formulated to treat acne skins. For details call Victoria Health on 0800 413596. To find a herbalist in your area for a tailor-made regimen, contact the **National Institute of Medical Herbalists** on 01392 426022.

Flower power Australian bush remedy combo: Spinifex, Five Corners, Billy Goat Plum. Spinifex has an internal cleansing action, Five Corners boosts self-confidence and Billy Goat Plum is the plant aborigine healers used to treat skin problems.

Anxiety and Embarrassment

What's happening?

Anxiety problems are the most common form of psychological

stress and can start as early as pre-teens. In its worst form, your child will get panic attacks and may even feel he or she is having a heart attack. Experts now believe that far from being all in the mind, a panic attack is the result of a malfunction in brain chemistry triggering the mind to send out the wrong signals at the wrong time. When anxiety is chronic, panic attacks are rare but the sufferer feels anxious most of the time. He or she may feel shy, embarrassed, uncomfortable and uneasy around other people and may suffer from regular headaches and even chronic fatigue (see page 54). Whatever the underlying causes, the following remedies can help.

What to do

Calcium is the 'tranquillizing' mineral – and if you are supplementing it, you need to give **magnesium** too (see Synergy, page 88) in a ratio of 2:1 in favour of the calcium. In acute cases, an underlying **iron deficiency** can increase the risk of a panic attack so make sure levels of this blood-building mineral are healthy too. All the **B vitamins** can reduce anxiety and soothe frazzled nerves. Give your child a good **B complex**. **Vitamin C** is also crucial for handling stress which could otherwise trigger acute anxiety. It is even more potent when combined with a bioflavonoid so for kids over five, give **Biocare's Children's Vitamin C and Bilberry**. Mail-order on 0121 433 3727.

The fastest-acting herbal remedy for anxiety is **kava kava**. (If you think 'calmer, calmer', you'll remember the name.) In any case, it should be called Chill Out, since that is just what the active ingredients – which are called pyrones – help the body to do. If you want the best results, buy the best product. **Lichtwer Pharma's Kava Kava** provides a standardized dose of the active ingredients and is backed by an impressive body of European research. You can contact the company direct on 01893 528668 or buy this brand in Boots.

Flower power Australian bush remedy combo: Confid Essence. This is the Australian bush combination remedy for shy kids (and mums). **Calm and Clear,** either in tincture or cream form, is excellent for youngsters with underlying anxiety. For an acute attack, use the **Emergency Essence** and cream. To learn more about flower remedies see page 124. For more information on the individual and combination ranges call Ancient Roots on 020 8421 9877 or visit the website at www.ancient-roots.com.

Asthma

What's happening?

The figures for childhood asthma have doubled in the last fifteen years – in some regions, as many as one in four children will now be asthmatic – and while we now know much more about the mechanism of asthma, nobody seems any closer to a cure.

What happens in children with asthma is that the airways narrow, making it much harder to breathe out, which then also restricts breathing in. This narrowing can be triggered by many everyday stimuli which don't have the same effect on the lungs and airways of a non-asthmatic. Among the more common triggers are house dust and animal hairs, but with your child the stimulus could just as easily be second-hand smoke, cold air or even exercise. You may also need to re-examine what is on the dinner plate. Many studies now indicate that food allergies are just as likely as environmental pollutants to trigger asthma in children. When researchers compared asthma rates among children living on the relatively unpolluted Isle of Skye with those living in mainland towns and cities, they found the incidence rate on the island much higher (17 per cent) than in Aberdeen or the national average, 11 per cent.

One unexpected new theory is that children eating more of the 'healthier' polyunsaturated fats (saturated fats are the ones found in meat and dairy products; polyunsaturated fats are found in margarines and some vegetable cooking oils) could be twice as much at risk. Australian researchers reporting the results of a 1,000-strong questionnaire in the medical journal *Thorax* also suggest that being breastfed offers more protection than being formula-fed. The survey raises more questions than it answers but the link between diet and asthma is now well established.

Anaphylaxis is the extreme allergic and sometimes fatal re-action to an allergen. New figures show the number of cases where this type of reaction is triggered by food is on the increase and that a key part of this life-threatening and extreme reaction is usually an asthmatic attack.

What to do

In one clinical study of asthmatic children, those given 1000mg of **vitamin C** each day for two weeks had less than a quarter as many asthmatic attacks as those given a placebo, making this a good starting point. **Vitamin B12**, particularly via intramuscular shots, has also been shown to dramatically reduce asthmatic symptoms. In another study of eighty-five patients, all sufferers benefited from a 1000mcg dose of B12 at weekly intervals and the younger the patient, the better the response, with 83 per cent of children under the age of ten showing marked improvement.

Homeopathic immunotherapy has also produced excellent clinical results in the treatment of asthma in children. In a French study of 182 children aged between two and eight, for example, the homeopathic remedy **Poumon histamine** was shown to reduce the number of severe asthma attacks. If you plan to take this route, find a qualified homeopath who can make a constitutional diagnosis of your child and prescribe accordingly. To find out how to get homeopathy on the NHS, contact the **British Homeopathic Association** on 020 7566 7800 and ask for the new patient guide booklet. This organization also keeps a list of doctors who are homeopaths too. To find other qualified homeopaths in your area, contact the **Society of Homeopaths** on 01604 621400.

Herbs can be useful too. **Lobelia extract**, for example, can help relieve an asthmatic attack, whatever is causing it (food, pollen or dust) because it works in the body to relax the smooth muscles of the bronchial airways. Keep a bottle of Napier's **Lobelia cough syrup** in the cupboard for emergencies but give as directed on the bottle and do not use internally for prolonged periods. (100ml costs £4.25. Mail-order on 0131 343 6683.) The **omega-6** and **omega-3 fatty acids** also work to keep airways clear. I like **Omega Nutrition's Essential Balance Jnr**, which is an organic, liquid formula from Higher Nature (01435 882880).

In Australia, where asthma rates are even higher than here, a natural remedy called **Oralmat,** which contains rye grass, has been shown to help asthma sufferers reduce the number and severity of attacks (see page 259). Oralmat, which is also reported to be effective against other allergies, colds, flu, respiratory problems, viral, fungal and bacterial infections, is now on sale in UK health stores. It costs £28 for 10ml. To give it, place three drops under the tongue. Keep the liquid there for fifteen seconds and then swallow. Repeat this three times a day. Mail-order from the Nutri Centre (020 7636 0422) if you cannot find it on the high street.

Flower power Australian bush remedy combo:* Red Grevillea,

---

*These remedies, remember, are not instead of other treatments but will work to support your child through an attack.

Grey Spider Flower, Little Flannel Flower, Bluebell. Red Grevillea for the feeling that something (the air) is stuck; Grey Spider Flower for the panic and terror of an acute attack; Little Flannel Flower for feeling smothered; Bluebell to open the heart chakra.

Athlete's Foot
(and other Fungal Infections)

What's happening?

Warm weather is usually the key trigger of fungal infections – especially athlete's foot – which is caused by one of two fungi, trichophyton or epidermophyton, both of which like to grow in the warm, moist areas between the toes. The trouble with over-the-counter remedies is that, while the problem appears to clear, reinfection is a problem.

Holistic practitioners take a more in-depth approach, which may include topical remedies to treat the symptoms, but which will also re-examine diet and lifestyle to identify the underlying causes. Since fungi are so common but not everyone develops an infection, complementary health practitioners interpret persistent fungal infections as a sign of (a) an imbalance in the body's microflora and (b) a weakened immune system.

What to do

Start from the inside out with a good quality **probiotic** to rebuild the protective bacteria in the gut (see page 95). To treat the skin topically, use a recommended **tea tree oil** product. A traditional antiseptic, it is five times stronger than any household detergent but completely safe to use on the skin. If using the pure oil, dilute it in a base oil before massaging onto the affected area. If this exacerbates the problem (by making that area more moist and greasy), abandon this and, instead, add six drops of the oil to warm water to make a foot bath to soak the affected area in. To support the immune system during an outbreak of fungal infection, use **echinacea** tincture.

Citricidal is another potent antifungal agent. Made from an extract of grapefruit seeds and widely on sale in health stores, it contains beneficial bioflavonoids, including a substance called **hesperidin** which is also a natural immune booster. As well as giving it internally as directed on the bottle, you can also apply it topically to the affected area.

If the infection persists, then switch to **colloidal silver**. A colloid is a substance that consists of ultra-fine particles suspended in a different medium (in this case, water). The particles are so small – 0.001 to 0.0001 of a micron in diameter – that colloidal silver is completely safe to use both internally and externally. Although nobody knows exactly how it works, the most accepted theory is that it disables the enzymes which many forms of bacteria, fungi and viruses need for their own metabolism and survival. While most antibiotics disinfect only about half a dozen germs, silver has been reported to disinfect well over 600 different strains. Even better, infections which can become resistant to antibiotics cannot develop the same defence against silver, making it an excellent alternative to antibiotics too. In fact, in more recent laboratory tests, scientists found colloidal silver was effective against many of the more insidious organisms that affect humans, including *Staphylococcus aureus*, *Salmonella typhi* and *Candida globata*.

Use **silica** to help prevent dampness and so change the conditions these fungi thrive on. It is best taken internally in the form of tissue salts which bypass the digestive system and so are more easily absorbed by the body.

Make a **red clover tea** and add it to the bathwater (see page 105).

Finally, use your common sense and **change the environment of the skin**. This could mean simply exposing the skin to fresh air and sunlight by wearing open-toed sandals, and making sure, after swimming, showering or taking a bath, that the skin between the toes is carefully dried with a towel nobody else will be using. Remember, these infections are highly contagious, and if you don't take care they will be passed back and forth within the family.

*****

Five-star Tip

To find out more about the health benefits of colloidal silver, the booklet *Colloidal Silver* by Zane Baranowski is excellent. It costs £2.99 and is available from the Nutri Centre bookshop (020 7436 5122).

Desert Essences specialize in tea tree oil remedies specifically for fungal infections, including athlete's foot. The relief spray costs £5.35. The cream is £4.99. A 30ml spray of colloidal silver made by **Source Naturals** costs £8.99. Silica No. 12 is a biochemic tissue salt made by **New Era** which costs £3.69. You can mail-order all these from Revital (0800 252875).

Flower power Australian bush remedy combo: Spinifex and Billy Goat Plum. Spinifex has a cleansing action on the skin and Billy Goat Plum will help clear any fungal infection.

Bed-wetting

What's happening?

Also known as nocturnal enuresis, bed-wetting which persists beyond the age of three is often linked with hidden allergies which can irritate the bladder, in some cases causing its walls to swell, thus reducing its capacity. The top five allergenic offenders are wheat, eggs, corn, milk and dairy products. Chocolate is an allergen too so temporarily eliminate all these to see if the problem resolves. If it does, then reintroduce them, one by one, to identify which ones are causing this problem. You may also find citrus fruits are triggering an allergic reaction in your child.

Bed-wetting is more common in boys and in children diagnosed as hyperactive, most of whom are boys too (see page 22). It can be the result of an underlying bladder infection or diabetes. If it persists, ask your doctor or health practitioner to check for these. Other common causes include emotional upsets, such as moving house or school or feeling insecure following the birth of a new baby. A viral infection, a common cold or, simply, a small bladder capacity may also be to blame. The bladder needs to be sufficiently big to hold the equivalent volume of one and a half cups of water to facilitate a dry night so if you are trying to cope with an immature bladder, avoid bedtime drinks. Make this a general rule for everyone to avoid making it seem as if the bed-wetting child is being punished for something he or she cannot control.

What to do

Avoid fizzy drinks – they stimulate the production of even more urine so save them for an occasional treat. **Constipation** may also put extra pressure on the bladder so make sure your child has regular and relaxed bowel movements (see page 314).

Minerals play a key role in keeping the bladder and urinary tract healthy – **sodium**, in particular, which is involved in regulating fluid levels in the body, can help with bladder problems. Buy a product that has been formulated for kids. I like **Biocare's**

Children's Multivitamin and Minerals, which is for kids aged two to twelve. Give children under four one capsule a day. If they can't swallow it, pierce the capsule with a sterile needle (heat it over a flame first) and add the liquid to a smoothie or fruit juice (for homemade Smoothies, see page 195).

Homeopathy gets excellent results in helping parents and their kids overcome this problem. Best is to consult a qualified homeopath. For over-the-counter remedies, try **Sepia 30x** or **9c** for children who typically wet the bed during the first two hours, and **Equisetum 30x** or **9c** for children who typically toss around all night and have active dreams and nightmares that wake them. Also try a combined Ura Ursi and oats remedy made by Bioforce and now widely on sale in health stores.

Unfortunately, one of the more common drugs given by modern medicine to treat bed-wetting is also used to help crack addicts get over their addiction to cocaine. A patient approach, using natural therapies, has to be a better long-term solution for a problem that only affects 10 per cent of children over five, most of whom will eventually grow out of it.

Flower power Australian bush remedy combo: Confid Combination essence and Bush Gardenia. If emotional problems and anxieties are to blame, give Confid Essence (see Anxiety, page 291). If there is a new baby or a new step-family, use Bush Gardenia, which works wonders with sibling rivalry.

Bites

What's happening?

You and the kids are awake half the night scratching at what turns out to be savage mosquito or other insect bites. You don't have to leave the UK to suffer – the horsefly bite can be just as bad as any mosquito, especially if anyone in the family has an allergic reaction.

What to do

You can prevent most bugs from biting in the first place by using **citronella**, **eucalyptus** or **lavender** oils. Remember, though, that essential oils should never be applied straight onto the skin. Dilute them first in a carrier oil such as almond (see page 119).

Researchers at the University of Glasgow who have been investigating the potent antimicrobial properties of an Indian herb called **neem** have now teamed up with the herbal medicine company Bioforce to develop a powerful insect repellent for use both at home and overseas. The scientists recently presented preliminary findings showing how neem, which is one of the most important medicinal plants to come out of India, reduced not only the number of mosquito bites but also the severity of the body's reaction so that both swelling and itching were lessened. How did they discover this? By sticking their hands into a laboratory tank of mosquitoes and waiting for the bites! If you cannot source the new repellent (which was not yet launched as we went to press) then invest instead in a bottle of the odd-smelling neem oil to massage onto the skin which will act in the same way. **Neem oil**, made from the seeds of the neem tree, costs £5.50 for 100ml. To mail-order and for stockist details of the pending repellent call Bioforce on 01294 277344.

If you are taking a break abroad, protect yourself and your family in advance by taking a supplement that combines the anti-inflammatory agent **quercetin** with **vitamin C**. One way this works is that quercetin helps stabilize the membranes of those cells that would otherwise discharge their supply of histamine into the surrounding blood and tissue when there is an allergic reaction to a bite. Vitamin C supports the immune system to improve the body's natural defences and also reduces the amount of histamine released. Activated **quercetin** made by **Natural Source** costs £12.99 for 50 capsules. Take 3–6 daily, between meals, and give the children an age-appropriate dose. If not available at your local health store, mail-order from Revital (0800 252875). To check safe dosages for kids, see page 65.

The herbalists and homeopaths at Farmacia have also formulated a new treatment cream called **Itch, Burn and Sting**. It contains nettle, calendula, rescue remedy and citronella oil and costs £4.95 for a 60g jar. Mail-order on 020 7831 0830.

Flower power Australian bush remedy combo: Emergency Essence Combination tincture and cream. Emergency Essence contains Fringed Violet to protect the body from all manner of attacks – physical and emotional. It is now sold as a cream (as well as a tincture), which you can use to treat insect bites.

Blisters

What's happening?

A blister is a build-up of fluid between layers of the skin and is usually a response to rubbing, friction, an allergy to an insect bite, an infection or a burn. The most important thing to do is to refrain from breaking open a blister, which will only worsen the infection.

As a kid I was quite an expert on blisters. Every summer I would start the holidays with brand-new blue rubber flip-flops and, within a day or two, had two sore blisters on each foot where the toe pieces had rubbed. In our gang you wore the flip-flops while the sores healed – it was a true badge of bravery and honour!

What to do

If a blister breaks open, wash the sore with diluted **tea tree oil** or **calendula cream**. Both will act as antiseptic agents. Then treat with comfrey salve. Mail-order **Burt's Bees Comfrey Salve** from Farmacia (020 7831 0830). An **aloe vera gel** can also help. If the blister remains sealed, you can try and draw the fluid out using a herbal compress (see page 107) made from **rosemary, witch hazel** or **yarrow**. For quality mail-order herbal suppliers, see page 108.

Flower power Australian bush remedy combo: Spinifex and Fringed Violet. Spinifex promotes cleansing and Fringed Violet supports the body while it recovers from injury and infection.

Broken Bones

What's happening?

A fractured bone can cause a limb to look crooked or bent and you may find your child lying perfectly still which is the body's own attempt to minimize the pain. The tissue around a broken bone will be very tender to the touch and may look red and swollen. Another problem with fractures is that the broken bone itself can damage other organs. A broken rib, for instance, can puncture a lung; a fracture to the skull could trigger bleeding into the brain. Any damage to the bone is traumatic and a serious shock to the whole body. If you suspect any kind of fracture, take your child to casualty immediately.

What to do

Once the bone has been X-rayed and re-set and your child is home, you can use herbs, homeopathy and nutrition to speed up the healing process.

Horsetail (*Equisteum arvense*) is rich in **silica**, a form of silicon and one of the trace elements that the body needs to make strong connective tissue. It also works in the body to improve the absorption of bone-building calcium from the diet. You can give silica on its own; the best form is **Biochemic Tissue Salts** which bypass the digestive system. Silica No. 12 is made by New Era and costs £3.69 from the Nutri Centre (020 7436 0422).

When you supplement the diet with **calcium**, remember you need to give **magnesium** too (see Synergy, page 88). The correct ratio is 2:1. Give one dose of 250mg of calcium with 125mg of magnesium, twice a day for two months. **Vitamin C** also plays a role in bone-healing so give a daily dose for at least three months after the break. A child recovering from a fracture should avoid fizzy drinks which leach phosphorus and calcium from the bones and weaken their structure.

Knitbone is the common name for **comfrey**, the other key herb which natural healers use to help mend broken bones. Comfrey contains rosmarinic acid which imparts anti-inflammatory properties but since it also contains alkaloids (which the body converts to toxic metabolites which have been linked to liver damage* in a handful of cases), the internal use of herbal medicines made from the root of the plant is now actively discouraged. The way around this is to use **Symphytum 6c** – the homeopathic version of comfrey – while the bone is still in plaster (and traction) and

---

*Other toxicity tests carried out on animals which suggested comfrey could cause cancer were later dismissed by experts who said that applying the same testing procedures would have proved carrots were carcinogenic too.

comfrey creams once the plaster is off and the wound has healed. If the bone is very slow to heal, you can give homeopathic **Calcium phosphate 6c** at night, along with the Symphytum, which you give in the morning. Continue with both remedies for two weeks. Weleda's Calcium phosphate 6c costs £3.50 for 125 tablets. Symphytum 6c from the same company costs the same. Granary Herbs make a comfrey cream which costs £3.25 for 50ml. All are available by mail order from Farmacia (020 7831 0830).

To treat a problem this serious, you should really be consulting a naturopath, who will know not to use a powdered form of comfrey for children. Instead, you will be advised to use a tincture where the active ingredients have been diluted down many times, or tablets where the dosage is standardized and you know exactly how much you are giving. To find a naturopath in your area, contact the **British Association of Nutritional Therapists** on 0870 606 1284. You will be charged £2 for a referral list. The **British Naturopathic Association** on 01458 840072 also holds a list of qualified naturopaths; it does not charge for referrals.

Flower power Australian bush remedy combo: Fringed Violet for the shock and **Red Helmet** to kick-start the body's own healing agents.

Bronchitis

What's happening?

This is a common and troublesome inflammation of the mucous membrane of the airways of the chest and lungs. Acute bronchitis is usually a viral infection. Less severe forms can be caused by bacteria and fungal infections. The tell-tale symptoms are a runny nose quickly followed by a dry, hacking cough which starts to produce phlegm after a few days. At this time, you may hear a rattling sound when your child breathes. Food allergies and intolerances, together with a compromised immune system, can make your child even more vulnerable so treatment should always start from the inside out. This condition, which can also be triggered by allergies – a cough that is worse at night is a sign of an allergic reaction – places the body under enormous stress and is often linked with a low-grade fever (see page 336).

What to do

If antibiotics have been prescribed, you will need to rebuild the good gut bacteria that aid digestion and the absorption of nutrients by supplementing the diet with a good quality probiotic. For children up to four, use **Solgar's ABC Dophilus powder** which costs £13.85 for 49.6g. For local stockists, call 01442 890355. For older kids use the new **Advanced Acidophilus Plus** (60 veggie capsules cost £7.95), Solgar's new generation probiotic made from two new strains of bacteria: *Lactobacillus acidophilus* LA5 and *Bifidobacterium lactus* BB12.

To help rebuild the immune system and to decongest the airways and keep them clear, use **Triton**, a new supplement made from three of the most powerful medicinal mushrooms known to man – **cordyceps** (*Cordyceps sinensis*), **reishi** (*Ganoderma lucidum*) and **shiitake** (*Lentinula edodes*), which work collectively to boost the immune system, increase aerobic performance and counter infection. This supplement contains 166mg of each mushroom and is sold in pots of 500mg tablets to last for six weeks (£18.95) or three months (£36). Mail-order from the UK specialists, Stewart Distribution, on 01273 558112. If swallowing tablets is a problem, crush them and sprinkle over cereals or spread with the butter in the lunchbox sandwich.

Eliminate mucus-forming foods from the diet. These include all high protein meats, high sugar foods and fried foods. In winter, serve chicken broth, which has been proved to reduce mucus, and make nourishing soups with carrots, which are rich in vitamin A which works to support mucous membranes in the body.

You can make your own **herbal cough syrup** by simmering equal parts of tincture of slippery elm, liquorice, marshmallow root and osha root in water. Add 40 drops of each herb in tincture form to 150ml/¼ pint water, simmer gently for 20 minutes, add honey to sweeten and give to your child when the mix has cooled. To save time, you can buy a good herbal mix from your local health store.

Finally, good old-fashioned **rest** is as important as any of the natural remedies you may be using. Allow younger children periods of moderate activity to prevent the secretions from settling and causing pneumonia; avoid contact with playmates to prevent the spread of the infection, and make sure your child drinks plenty of fluids in the form of water, homemade fruit juices and soothing herbal teas.

Flower power Australian bush remedy: Dagger Hakea, the remedy for both respiratory problems and underlying emotional resentments.

Bruises

What's happening?

Have you ever wondered what a bruise actually is? It's a pool of blood that has escaped from its blood vessels following an injury to one of the tiny capillaries close to the surface of the skin, caused by a bump, thump, bang or fall at that site. This blood becomes trapped under the skin, causing the familiar discoloration of a bruise which disappears as the body reabsorbs the leaking blood. Any new bruise will feel tender and may be swollen too. The reason bruises sometimes look brown or yellow as they heal is that, as the fluids are reabsorbed, a little residual iron from the blood may be left over.

What to do

If you have younger or accident-prone kids, never leave home without a small tube of **arnica cream** which you can use for all types of bruises, strains, sprains and swellings. I use **Weleda's** cream which is on sale now in all good high street health stores. I also keep a handy supply of high potency homeopathic **Arnica 30c** for emergencies. If you are tackling bruising that is the result of surgery, give this high potency remedy two days before the operation and continue for two days afterwards. Give four little pills of Arnica 30c at night and in the morning, and again just before surgery. Remember to tip these from the container under the tongue and to avoid touching them, which can contaminate the active ingredient.

A child who bruises very easily may be deficient in vitamin C, bioflavonoids and vitamin K (see Supplements, page 64). The first two of these nutrients are involved in building strong blood vessels and the latter, vitamin K, plays a key role in blood-clotting. **Biocare's Children's Vitamin C and Bilberry** (the latter is a bioflavonoid and these two nutrients are synergistic) is formulated for children aged five and over. To mail-order call 0121 433 3727. For age-related doses, see page 65.

If you are on the spot to deal with a bruise immediately, apply **ice** or a **cold compress** (see page 107) to the affected area. If using ice, be sure to protect the skin by wrapping the ice first in a clean cloth which will form a barrier and prevent any frostbite damage.

Flower power Australian bush remedy combo: Five Corners encourages your child to take more care of him or herself as he or she charges around and **Flannel Flower** boosts energy to help physical recovery.

Chicken Pox

What's happening?

Few children escape childhood without succumbing to this highly contagious infection – which is probably just as well since the adult version is so much more dangerous. Caused by the varicella-zoster virus, which is a relation of the herpes family, it usually starts with a headache, tiredness, loss of appetite and a fever. After a day or two, the tell-tale rash of spots will appear. The important thing to remember is that an infected child is contagious from up to forty-eight hours before the first symptoms appear until all of the blisters are dry and scabbed over. The more intimate and more frequent the exposure to this virus, the more severe the infection will be. This means that if the condition is running through the family, children who are at different stages of the disease need to be kept apart.

Spot-the-rash: it first appears as a flat, reddish rash which then turns into clusters of tiny pimples and blisters that crust over as they heal. In most cases, the rash starts on the torso and spreads to the outer limbs. There are usually few blisters on the head or neck but those that do appear elsewhere on the body are horribly itchy.

What to do

Keep your child well hydrated by making sure he or she drinks plenty of fluids. Serve simple and nutritious dishes such as chicken broth, light vegetable soups and well-cooked grains. If your child cannot face eating, make fruit popsicle lollies.

Vitamin A is key to skin healing and can be given as a supplement in its own right (see page 66 for doses), or you can use **betacarotenes** which the body then converts to vitamin A.

Traditional herbalists use **blessed thistle** (*Cnicus benedictus*) to reduce fever in both chicken pox and measles. It is rich in skin-healing vitamin A, immune-boosting zinc and the stress-busting B vitamins. To mail-order supplies, call Herbs of Grace (01638 750140), and use as directed.

A herbal mix of **echinacea** and **goldenseal** will give any viral infection a battering. As well as boosting immunity, this mighty antiviral combination will also help clear the infection and accelerate tissue healing. To treat the lesions, use superstrength manuka honey. New from Comvita, **Active UMF10 Manuka** will promote healing and prevent secondary infection. The 10 is a potency ranking and UMF stands for Unique Manuka Factor. This superstrength honey costs £11.50 for a 375g jar. (For mail order see page 312.) Use a sterile swab to gently dab the healing blisters. Use diluted Bergamot oil in the same way.

Soothe frazzled nerves (yours and theirs) and an irritable child with **chamomile tea** which you can serve lukewarm to older kids or frozen in popsicle form. A mild **lavender milk bath** can also help relieve some of the itching and irritation of the sores. Once the sores have healed and the scabs have gone, massage a good quality rose oil or rosa mosqueta into the affected area to prevent scarring. I use Living Nature's fabulous **Rose and Herbs Oil** (mail-order on 01489 56614) or **Rosa Mosqueta** from Rio Trading (01273 0570987).

Trying to stop a child itching is a parent's nightmare. Homeopathic **calendula** in tincture, oil or gel form can take the sting out of the urge to scratch. For intense itching, use homeopathic **Rhus toxicodendron**. Give a 30x or 9c potency, three times a day until the symptoms improve. For the best results with homeopathy, consult a qualified practitioner.

Flower power Australian bush remedy combo: Black-eyed Susan and Red Grevillea – stops itching and supports the body through the stress of a viral infection.

Cold Sores

What's happening?

Cold sores are caused by the herpes simplex virus 1 (HSV-1) which is related to but not the same as the virus that causes genital herpes. The sores first appear up to ten days after initial exposure to the virus, which then remains in the system for ever. Up to 60 per cent of children have this virus by the age of ten and although it will remain mostly dormant, common triggers include stress, sunlight, fever, tiredness or too much white sugar.

The cold sore virus is also activated by an amino acid called arginine. Foods that are rich in arginine and which your child needs to avoid include chocolate, nuts – such as peanut butter – and most cereal grains. A second amino acid called lysine works to inhibit the absorption of arginine and therefore helps suppress this virus. Natural sources of virus-suppressing lysine include dairy products and potatoes, so unless there is an underlying dairy intolerance, serve more of these foods.

What to do

Recurrent cold sores signal that the immune system is weakened. Build it up again with foods that are rich in **zinc,** including eggs, turkey and sunflower or pumpkin seeds. (Disguise the latter by blending a tablespoon with salad dressings or in smoothies and see Immune System, page 268.) Give your child a **lysine supplement** (250mg, three times a day). Foods that are high in lysine will also help. As well as dairy, these include tuna, salmon and wholemeal bread.

Treat the sores with antiviral **grapefruit seed extract** or dab with **manuka honey.** Buy the superstrength **UMF10 Manuka** from **Comvita.** UMF stands for Unique Manuka Factor and is a newly introduced scheme to grade potency. UMF10 is the grade used in hospitals to treat wounds and sores. (375g costs £11.50. Mail-order direct on 01730 813642.) Treat outbreaks overnight with pure **tea tree oil** (I use the Desert Essence brand) which will reduce the severity and duration of an infection.

To prevent re-infection, keep a bottle of **Elagen** in the bathroom cupboard. The active ingredient is an Asian plant called *Eleutherococcus senticosus* which is related to immune-boosting ginseng and safe to give to children.

Lysine supplements and grapefruit seed lotions are on sale in good health stores. Elagen costs £11.35 for 30 capsules and is available by mail order from a company called Eladon in Bangor, Wales (01248 370059).

Flower power Australian bush remedy combo: Spinifex, Sturt Desert Rose, Billy Goat Plum. Spinifex has a cleansing action in the body and is brilliant for healing skin lesions. Sturt Desert Rose promotes a more positive acceptance of the body with all its faults and flaws, and Billy Goat Plum can eliminate those feelings of disgust which accompany an outbreak of this infection.

Colic

What's happening?

If you have a baby who won't stop crying, the chances are your family and friends will have already diagnosed colic. The word 'colic' comes from the Greek word for the large intestine, telling us that although nobody really knows the underlying causes, this is believed to be linked back to a digestive disorder. In fact, even though there has never been any proof, most people accept it is a distressing sign of cramping abdominal pain and gas.

Colic is most common in the first three weeks to six months of life. It is rare for a baby older than this still to be suffering. For distraught parents, the single defining factor is that no matter what you do, the crying doesn't stop and the baby is inconsolable.

What to do

Researchers at the Department of Experimental Research at the University of Lund in Sweden report that a quarter of all babies with mild to moderate colic are reacting to cow's milk. They pinpointed several signs of abnormal intestine function in colicky infants and recommended that breastfeeding mothers **adopt a strict dairy-free diet** for themselves and take calcium supplements instead. Formula-fed infants should also be taken off cow's milk and given a hypoallergenic, casein-hydrolysate formula.

Mothers are also told to hold and carry their colicky babies in a bid to comfort them but Dutch doctors conducting a review of the effectiveness of current treatments for colic reported that not only does this fail to reduce the crying, this extra stimulation can sometimes make it worse.

Breastfeeding mothers can drink soothing herbal teas which will pass through the breast to the baby. The best ones are **fennel** and **lemon balm** (to find out how to make herbal teas, see page 106). You can also help relieve abdominal spasms by giving baby a warm bath using safe herbal flower waters or bath milks (see Essential Oils, page 119). To make a lavender bath milk add 1 drop of the essential oil to 20ml (a generous tablespoon) of full-fat milk and add to the bath water.

The best excuse ever . . . not to eat your greens! Between three and six months, other foods that the mother may be eating can also trigger colic in breastfed babies. The worst culprits include: chocolate, coffee, spicy foods, curries, garlic, onions, alcohol, broccoli, cabbage, beans, legumes, cauliflower, Brussels sprouts, grapes, peaches, plums, strawberries and pineapple. Dairy products are a trigger at all ages.

Flower power Australian bush remedy combo: Black-eyed Susan and Emergency Essence. Black-eyed Susan supports all the body's systems through extra stress; Emergency Essence can relieve panic and pain.

Constipation

What's happening?

If your child complains of difficulty in passing stools, then he or she is suffering from constipation, which in kids can be a sign of insufficient vitamin C and magnesium in the diet. If you are giving vitamin C supplements to very young kids, choose a buffered form such as ascorbate. Your first step, though, must be to increase these two nutrients in the diet by persuading them to eat more foods that are rich in both, especially dark leafy greens, broccoli, dried apricots and seafoods.

Fresh vegetable juices will also help clear the large intestine. If your children will eat them, juice fresh kiwi fruits, which contain more vitamin C than oranges, and increase their intake of all fluids with lots of fresh homemade juices, water and herbal teas to help soften hard stools.

Lots of children will resist the urge to go to the lavatory through idleness or because they are preoccupied, so watch out for this. Also, once constipation is already causing some discomfort, your child may procrastinate even more. Try to actively encourage more regular bowel habits (such as going to the lavatory at the same time each day) and with younger children build in lots of free time for running around and letting off steam since this kind of exercise will promote a good flow of blood to the colon to help keep it in good working order.

What to do

The herbs **marshmallow** and **slippery elm** are both excellent natural and gentle laxatives which are safe to give to children in the correct dosages (see page 101). They work because they are high in mucilage – a substance that combines with water in the colon to develop a gel-like consistency which then softens the stools.

If the bowel is cramping, causing stomach pains, make a warm **chamomile** tea or buy it in tincture form. **Ginger**, in juices or tincture form, can also ease digestion and stop painful spasms.

Once you have kick-started the peristaltic wave action of the colon that eliminates waste from the body, you need to keep it working optimally by avoiding too many of the foods which slow down this action. The worst offenders are animal products, especially meat, cheese and milk. Homemade nut milks are an excellent substitute, as long as there is no underlying nut allergy.

To make these, simply grind your chosen nuts in a blender and collect the liquid.

For older kids, you can sprinkle **organic flaxseed** on breakfast cereals to increase the right kind of fibre in the diet, but if this causes a commotion, slip **flaxseed oil** into smoothies instead. This is better than using wheat bran, which can irritate a sensitive gut wall. For younger children (up to 2 years old), stick to Solgar's **ABC Dophilus powder** which costs £13.85 for 49.6g and which you need to keep in the fridge. For local stockists, call 01442 890355.

The best prebiotic on sale in health stores is still **FOS** which is sold in powdered form too. The sweeter the taste, the higher the purity, so check before you buy. Add to smoothies or breakfast cereals. You can mail-order **FOS powder** (250g costs £6.10) from Revital (0800 252875). Add £1.50 p&p.

For older kids, **Nutrition Now's Rhino FOS and Acidophilus** combines pre- and probiotics in an additive-free supplement powder. Mail-order from Victoria Health on 0800 413596 and add 1 teaspoon a day to food or juices. For teens and adults, **PB 8** from the same company contains not two, not four, but eight different strains of good bacteria to aid digestion.

The human body was never designed for the modern lavatory, so, if you have teens complaining of constipation, keep a footstool or child's step in the bathroom. Explain how, by placing the feet on this stool while seated on the lavatory, it puts the body in a more natural position to evacuate the bowels and reduces any element of straining.

Flower power Australian bush remedy combo: Bluebell, Bottlebrush and Boronia. Bottlebrush supports the natural systems of the body; Boronia can counter a feeling of 'fullness', and Bluebell is all about releasing feelings which have been 'suppressed'.

Coughs, Colds and Flu

Coughs: What's happening?

Coughing is a natural reflex mechanism used to clear foreign bodies from the respiratory passages. However, there are many different types of coughs in response to a multitude of triggers so you need to work out what you are dealing with.

A dry and irritating cough, for instance, can be due to infection in the nose, sinus, ear or throat, or may be provoked by inhaling second-hand cigarette smoke. A loose and wet cough may be a sign of bronchitis (see page 305) or triggered by an allergy. A cough which worsens at night is usually a sign of inflammation and the result of a shift in fluids, caused by lying down, which then triggers the cough reflex.

What to do

If your child has a productive cough, it is important to reduce the production of mucus in the body. This means ruling out the high protein, high mucus-forming foods such as red meat and dairy produce for a while. Don't think switching to soy products is the answer because these are high in protein too and so have the same action in the body. If you are worried about your child getting enough calcium when dairy is off the menu, give them a supplement (see page 78).

Chicken broth helps to 'thin' existing mucus and is a good example of the more nourishing foods you should be giving to a child who has a cough or cold. If the family is vegetarian, choose highly coloured vegetables which are rich in the betacarotenes and bioflavonoids that help the body make **vitamin A,** to soothe its mucous membranes. These also enhance the immune-supporting activity of other nutrients such as **vitamin C** and **zinc**. **Nutri's Echinacea ACZ** provides all three nutrients – vitamins A, C and zinc, plus betacarotenes. It costs £14.50 for 60 capsules. Mail-order from the Nutri Centre on 020 7436 5122. Or you can order online at www.nutricentre.com.

Napier's Lobelia cough syrup will help dislodge mucus. Formulated by medical herbalists, it costs £4.24 for 100ml and works because the active ingredient, an alkaloid called lobeline, stimulates the respiratory tract. To mail-order, call 0131 343 6683. The new **Boots Alternatives** range also includes a **Breathe Easy Rub** which blends **grapefruit, eucalyptus** and **peppermint oils** and which is safe to gently massage over the upper chest and throat at bedtime.

Colds: What's happening?

A cold is a viral infection of the upper respiratory tract and while a healthy adult catches just two colds a year, children can get between six and nine. The well-recognized symptoms can include a runny or blocked nose, sneezing, a headache, a sore throat, coughing, loss of appetite, streaming eyes, ear congestion, a low-grade fever, and aching muscles and joints.

What is happening is that as the virus multiplies, the mucous membranes in the respiratory tract become swollen and increase mucus production which, in turn, narrows the airways, making breathing more difficult. A typical cold will run for around ten days, but if the child's temperature reaches 38.8°C/102°F, you are dealing with the flu.

What to do

Since children, like adults, are more at risk when feeling tired or run down, it makes sense to support their immune system through winter to reduce the risk of catching a cold. Support a child's still immature immune system by supplementing the diet with **vitamin C** combined with a **bioflavonoid** such as **rosehip** or **quercetin** plus **betacarotenes** and **zinc**.

Ginger tea will warm the body, increase perspiration and help reduce the intensity of a heavy cold. **Sage tea** will break down mucus congestion but is an acquired taste, even for older kids. If you are using herbal teas, give one cup three times a day for between three and five days. The moment you suspect a child is succumbing to a cold, give a combined **goldenseal** and **echinacea** treatment. You can mix tinctures of both herbs or use a ready-made formula.

If you don't have time to make your own herbal popsicles (see page 108), **Goodypops** are an ingenious way to get your kids to take the herbs and nutrients that will protect them from coughs and colds over winter. The Goodypops lolly will not only soothe a sore throat, but boost the immune system too. It combines vitamin C with echinacea which has now been shown in clinical trials to increase the number of white blood cells, the body's first defence against disease. There are two lollipop flavours – banana honey and field berry. Both also contain pectin, a natural substance found in citrus fruits which works in the body to soothe and coat the throat. Goodypops are sold in packs of eight which cost £1.95 and are on sale in high street health shops.

Flu: What's happening?

Anyone who has ever had flu can tell you just how miserable the symptoms make you feel. This is a viral infection and because the virus is clever enough to change its structure every couple of years, nobody can build a lifelong immunity following an infection. In other words, your family is always at risk of catching one of the newer strains.

What to do

Since the typical symptoms are chills, fever, headache, achiness, fatigue and no appetite, the key to managing them lies in controlling the fever, getting plenty of rest and keeping the body well hydrated with healthy fluids.

New to the UK (and my household this past winter) is **Sambucol,** a range of potent antiviral products made from one of nature's oldest remedies, **black elderberries** (*Sambucus nigra*). Developed by Dr Madeleine Mumcuoglu Ph.D., a virologist who lost both her paternal and maternal grandmothers to influenza in the 1950s, it works by attacking and deactivating the virus before it can spread its invasion throughout the body. Researchers at the Department of Virology at the Hebrew University Hadassah Medical School in Jerusalem have conducted preliminary clinical trials on the range and reported excellent recovery rates. In a survey of forty flu patients, they found those taking Sambucol recovered twice as quickly as those given a placebo. The scientists concluded that the active ingredient of the black elderberry could shorten the duration of a flu attack to just four days. **Sambucol for Kids** includes vitamin C and bee propolis and actually tastes quite nice. Mail-order from Higher Nature (01435 882964). Give as directed on the bottle at the first signs of an infection.

Flower power Australian bush remedy combo: For colds and flu combine **Paw Paw, Black-eyed Susan** and **Jacaranda** to keep the body strong. For coughs use **Illawarra Flame Tree**, **Dagger Hakea** and **Red Helmet** to clear the airways.

Cradle Cap

What's happening?

When the sebum-producing oil glands in the scalp go into overdrive, you will see the tell-tale sign of cradle cap, a thick, waxy, yellowish encrustation most prevalent at the top of your baby's head. A form of seborrhoeic dermatitis, which is an inflammatory skin complaint, it can also appear on the eyebrows and eyelids, in and around the ears, around the nose and in the groin area. This is a classic Catch 22 problem because when excess oil starts to flake, it clogs the ducts of the glands, which respond by producing even more oil in an attempt to unblock the plug and clear the pathway to the surface. And then you get deeper plugs, even more waxy scales and even more oil production. Cradle cap looks very itchy but is not. Your biggest problem is making sure a secondary bacterial or fungal infection does not spot its opportunity to take hold.

What to do

To reduce the risk of fungal infections, build the good bacteria in your baby's system by supplementing the diet with an infant probiotic. **Biocare's Bifidobacterium Infantis** is safe for newborns and older. It costs £22.50 for 60g. Mail-order direct from the company on 0121 433 3727 and mix a quarter of a teaspoon with a little warm water daily.

Mix a little **olive oil** and pure **tea tree oil** (I use the Desert

Essence brand which is about as pure as you can get) and massage affected areas with this lotion. Then shampoo and brush the greasy scale away. Washing your baby's hair every day is not enough to clear cradle cap – this is not a problem caused by poor hygiene – and so to help unplug the blocked ducts, you will need to brush the scalp firmly with a soft baby brush. Never pick at any lesions, which could trigger an infection. When you do shampoo, make sure you are using a shampoo that does not contain sodium lauryl sulphate – a foaming agent which, in high concentrations, can lead to the breakdown of protein in the body.

Always be on guard against infection. If you spot any affected area that looks red and feels warm to the touch, or if you notice an unusual discharge, consult a qualified health practitioner – a naturopath, homeopath or your doctor.

Flower power Australian bush remedy: Billy Goat Plum, to promote healthy skin.

Cuts and Scrapes

What's happening?

A deep and gaping cut is going to need medical treatment, maybe even stitches, but the minor wounds and grazes that are an inevitable part of an active childhood can be safely treated at home with natural remedies that can help relieve the pain, prevent infection, promote rapid tissue healing and minimize scarring.

What to do

The first thing you need to do with an open wound is to clean and disinfect it to prevent infection. Wash with diluted **tea tree oil** but use a brand that is pure and high in the active ingredients. The Desert Essence brand, which is now widely on sale, is eco-harvested, 100 per cent organic and as pure as you can get. (For local stockists, call 020 8614 1411.)

Manuka honey is harvested in New Zealand from bees feasting on the pollen of the tea tree and is such a powerful healing agent it has now been licensed for medical use in hospitals throughout Australia. Makers have introduced a new Unique Manuka Factor (UMF) potency scale so look for a product that has a UMF of 10 or more. I use this when there is no need to cover the wound. **Calendula cream** is another excellent antiseptic lotion for minor cuts and grazes. Mail-order from Napiers (0131 343 6683).

Organic sulphur – sold as **MSM** which is short for methyl-sulphonylmethane – promotes tissue healing from the inside. This nutrient plays a key role in making collagen, the primary component of cartilage and connective tissue. It is present in cow's milk and fresh fruits, as well as meat and seafoods, but is easily destroyed by cooking so supplementation is a safer bet. Higher Nature sells MSM powder, tablets and creams. For details, call 01435 882964.

Rosa mosqueta oil from South America was originally developed as an antiwrinkle skin cream but holistic skin therapists were soon reporting back on its ability to significantly reduce scarring. Their empirical findings have now been corroborated by Chilean researchers at the University of Concepcion who confirmed its incredible skin regenerative properties after treating 180 patients presenting with surgical or burn scars. Sales of rosa mosqueta are currently worth more than US$30 million to Chile. In the UK, you can mail-order the oil from Rio Trading on 01273 570987. A 20ml bottle costs £9.99. Do not massage onto the affected area until the wound has healed.

Flower power Australian bush remedy combo: Give **Emergency**

Essence which combines Fringed Violet, Grey Spider Flower and Dog Rose for the shock, Crowea to help regain balance and Warratah for courage.

Diarrhoea

What's happening?

If you think about it, diarrhoea is simply the body's fast-track way of getting rid of toxins and other harmful substances, so rather than trying to stop it, the more holistic approach is to support your child while his or her body cleanses itself and, most importantly, to make sure he or she stays hydrated by drinking lots of fluids.

Of all the underlying reasons for a sudden onset of diarrhoea, food poisoning is one of the biggest culprits, but your child may also have a viral or bacterial infection picked up from another child at school or outside the home. Food intolerances can cause diarrhoea in younger kids so if you've introduced a new food and witnessed this reaction, you can make the link for yourself. Less common causes include inflammatory bowel disorders, coeliac disease, hepatitis, cystic fibrosis or an anatomical problem with the gut. If you suspect any of these, see your doctor right away. If you have an infant who develops diarrhoea, call your health visitor or local surgery.

In most cases, though, diarrhoea is being caused by a viral infection of the intestinal tract which becomes irritated and inflamed. The virus triggers the cells lining the intestines to secrete more fluids. This intensifies the peristaltic or wave-like action of the gut which moves food along and then you have a child with painful stomach cramps and loose, watery and frequent stools.

What to do

Prevent dehydration by persuading your child to take **small, frequent sips of filtered water**. Do not encourage gulping large quantities of fluids, which could cause vomiting. If vomiting does occur, have your child suck ice cubes instead.

If your child wants to eat, serve small, light and nourishing meals such as homemade soups and broths. From the onset of symptoms, **cut out all dairy products** and do not reintroduce for a fortnight, which will give the gut time to heal. **Avoid protein** for two days to give the digestive tract a rest, and eliminate all hard-to-digest fats until symptoms have disappeared.

Give a child-friendly **probiotic** to redress the balance of good and bad bacteria in the gut and mix powdered **slippery elm** with a little apple juice and water to make a herbal paste that will soothe the infected lining of the gut. **Biocare's Strawberry or Banana-flavoured Acidophilus** is excellent for kids over the age of six months. Mail-order on 0121 433 3727. You can buy slippery elm from Napiers on 0131 343 6683: 95g costs £6.05.

Repeated bouts of diarrhoea may be a sign of lactose intolerance. See page 349.

Flower power Australian bush remedy: Paw Paw supports the body as it struggles to clear out an infection.

Dyslexia

What's happening?

Everyone knows someone who's dyslexic but lots of us make the mistake of thinking this condition is only about reading difficulties. In fact, it's a recognized neurodevelopmental syndrome whose features can include memory weakness and difficulty with direction and sequencing, as well as letters which jump and jiggle and dance about the page. Slow or abnormal spoken language development is an early sign of this condition which, in its most severe form, affects some 5 per cent of the general population and many more males than females.

What to do

Arginine is an amino acid which is sold in supplement form as L-arginine. It has a similar action in the body to a prescription drug called piracetam, which has been shown in trials to facilitate learning and memory. Both the drug and arginine are believed to have some effect on the fluidity of the membrane barrier that surrounds and protects the brain, allowing only certain nutrients and chemicals to pass through. That said, until someone carries out widescale clinical trials, these claims will remain speculative.

What neuroscientists do now agree on is that this condition, along with behavioural disorders such as dyspraxia, ADD and ADHD (see pages 22–7) may be linked back to a problem in metabolizing fatty acids in the body and that the solution, for some families, will be as simple as supplementing the diet with a high dose (2 tablespoons/30ml or the equivalent of 1g) of highly unsaturated fatty acids (**HUFA**s). These can be sourced from foods such as oily fish and nuts (as long as there is no underlying allergy) but not in high enough doses to make a real difference.

Researchers now believe at least a third of all children with neurodevelopmental disorders, including dyslexia, may be deficient in these important nutrients. Key signs that your dyslexic child may be among this group include dry skin and hair, soft or brittle nails, excessive thirst, frequent urination and dandruff. Follicular keratosis, where patches of skin become 'dry and bumpy', may be another sign. One of the best blends of the essential fatty acids that the body cannot make but must get from the diet is **Udo's Choice**, formulated by the world-famous fat expert Udo Erasmus. Sourced from flaxseed, sunflower, sesame seed, evening primrose, rice bran and oat bran oils, it is widely on sale in high-street health stores where 250ml costs around £8.95. If you prefer an organic product, **Omega Nutrition's Essential Balance Jnr** is also excellent and, since it tastes of butterscotch, probably easier to slip into food. If you can't find it locally, mail-order from Higher Nature on 01435 882880.

Rhino Actalin from **Nutrition Now** contains phosphatidyl-choline (see page 241), a form of the brain chemical choline which works to repair the membranes of nerve cells and stimulate the utilization of fatty acids. Described on the bottle as providing 'brain support' it costs £12.65 for 60 chewable tablets, and in the UK is available only from Victoria Health (0800 413596).

Flower power Australian bush remedy combo: Bush Fuchsia, Sundew and Jacaranda: This tailor-made combination promotes learning and helps kids stay focused in class.

Ear Infections

What's happening?

An ear infection is frequently the first sign that a child is sickening for something and by the age of three, almost all children will have succumbed to some type of inner ear infection. An allergic reaction to certain foods, especially dairy products, can cause an infection in the outer ear (external otitis) but far more common in infants and children is an infection of the inner ear (otitis media) caused by bacteria or viruses. Ear infections are also often a complication of a cold or other respiratory problem and may be accompanied by a runny nose and sore throat.*

What to do

The conventional treatment is antibiotics and if you take this route, make sure you support your child's gut flora by giving him or her a good quality **probiotic** (see page 95). **Zinc** will boost the immune system and one of the best ways to give this mineral to younger kids is via throat lozenges. **Nature's Plus Kids' Zinc Lozenges** combine immune-boosting zinc with echinacea, olive leaf extract and ginger: 60 tablets cost £7.49. Mail-order from Revital (0800 252875).

You've heard of **echinacea** – the top-selling immune-boosting herb – but you may not have come across **plantago,** which partners it in a brand new Bioforce tincture formulated to treat ear infections in kids. Plantago is an odourless plant found in Europe and Asia where it grows in vast quantities in dry meadows and fields. It has both astringent and expectorant properties, which have made it a traditional treatment for bronchial infections and infections of the nasal passages, as well as inflammation of the inner ear. Its soothing action is thanks to the high proportion of mucilage found in the plant. **Bioforce's Echinacea Complex** is a herbal tincture that includes plantago. It costs £4.79 for 30ml. To mail-order call 01294 277344.

Recent reports suggesting that of the eleven varieties of echinacea, *Echinacea angustifolia* is the most potent are rubbish. Independent tests show it is not more active than the more widely used *Echinacea purpurea*. You may also read or be told it is 'unsafe' to use echinacea for longer than two weeks. Again, this

---

* If your child complains of chills, dizziness and hearing loss, go to your doctor.

has now been shown to be wrong. You can use the herb for as long as you need to.

You can also clear an ear infection by gently putting 2–4 drops of warmed **liquid garlic** in each ear. Make sure that you use a different dropper for each ear, to stop the spread of infection.

Flower power Australian bush remedy combo: Kangaroo Paw and Bush Gardenia. These are the remedies for all ear problems. Bush Gardenia is also the essence for family bonds.

Eczema

What's happening?

Also known as atopic dermatitis, this is one of the most common childhood complaints. Eczema is always an allergic response to an allergen, which may be a food or some other everyday item such as a household detergent that has come into contact with the skin. In children, **allergies to milk, eggs and peanuts** account for over 80 per cent of eczema cases – all believed to be caused by an underlying condition known as **leaky gut** (see page 170). There is usually a strong family history of eczema and most sufferers go on to develop asthma or hay fever or both.

Infants with eczema are usually reacting to something in the breastmilk and the mother's diet, and here, again, eczema is generally a sign of a problem with digestion. An overgrowth of the yeast candida albicans (see page 387), which is very common after a course of antibiotics, is also linked with this skin complaint, which is characterized by an itchy, red and inflamed rash that can appear anywhere on the body. The rash may be dry, scaly and cracked, which will cause the skin to thicken, or wet, weepy and oozing.

What to do

Remove dairy and peanut products and eggs from the diet and see if this has any effect on the skin. Avoid all foods with additives and preservatives (see page 34) and steer clear of refined sugar. In some kids, **wheat** may be causing a problem too so look for alternatives (see page 169) and monitor the response. Allow 6–8 weeks for these dietary changes to take effect.

Once you have identified and eliminated food or chemical triggers, concentrate on rebuilding a strong immune system and digestive tract. **Calendula**, which has anti-inflammatory properties, and **echinacea**, which can boost immunity, both work well to build a child's natural defences and are widely available in health stores now. Tinctures act faster than capsules but the dosage is more hit-and-miss so once the rash has cleared, switch to a supplement that tells you how much of the active ingredient you are getting. (See page 101 for safe herbal dosages.)

To rebuild strong digestion, supplement the diet with a good quality **probiotic** (see page 95). If you are using a probiotic powder for infants, give half a teaspoon a day, mixed with a little warm water.

Essential fatty acids, which the body cannot make but must glean from the diet, also help. Researchers report that eczema sufferers cannot process fatty acids, which can result in a deficiency in gammalinoleic acid (GLA). **Evening primrose oil** can remedy this and in double-blind, placebo-controlled clinical trials was shown to dramatically reduce itching. The researchers were using high doses – the equivalent of 45mg of GLA a day. You can also use **fish oils** (1–3 teaspoons a day) or, if you prefer a vegetarian option, **flaxseed oil**, but you need to keep using the oil of your choice for six months to a year.

Living Nature's Eczema Kit includes evening primrose oil to be taken internally, a Manuka cleansing gel, a hand and body cream for dry eczema and one for wet eczema, plus an eczema information sheet. It costs £28.60. For more information, call 01489 566144.

For general skincare, the **Botanicals Therapeutic** range, which includes shampoos, soaps and skin lotions, can help soothe and control eczema. For details, call Victoria Health on 0800 413596. If you are dealing with a chronic case, you can't beat the natural skin therapists at **The Alternative Centre** (020 7381 2298) in London who specialize in treating eczema and psoriasis in all ages.

To find out how other eczema sufferers – kids, their parents and adult sufferers – cope with the condition, check out a new website called www.eczemavoice.com.

*****

Five-star Tip

SK Cream for eczema is one of those secret, word-of-mouth remedies that people only tell their relatives and friends about. Developed quietly by a family of organic farmers to treat their relatives, it worked so well they now ship some 20,000 tubs to 20 different countries. The organic formula includes chamomile, almond oil and beeswax and there is a lanolin-free version for anyone allergic to this substance. A 30ml jar costs £9.95 including p&p. To mail-order call 01526 832491 but remember, this is a kitchen table (actually a cow barn) business with only one order line so be patient if you cannot get through the first time you call.

Flower power Australian bush remedy combo: Dagger Hakea and Billy Goat Plum. Emotional upsets will often trigger an outbreak so keep these Australian bush remedies – which tackle resentment and promote healthy skin – in the bathroom cupboard at all times.

Endometriosis

What's happening?

Endometriosis is another of those mostly hidden conditions that have doctors foxed. Although it runs in families, nobody really knows what causes it or why some females will have only a mild form of the disease but suffer excruciating symptoms, while others will have a severe form but report no symptoms at all.

What happens is that the same sort of cells that grow normally in the lining of the womb begin to grow outside the uterus. One theory is that these cells actually migrate from the uterus. Another is that they are different types of cell that have mutated due to an error in their genetic programming.

The most likely sites for endometriosis to occur are the ovaries, the Fallopian tubes, the bladder and the bowel, and although more common in older females, it can occur in girls as young as fifteen who will struggle through their teens with painful periods and no serious diagnosis of the problem. Symptoms range from painful periods to infertility and, in extreme cases, major surgery to cut away these patches of tissue is the last resort.

What to do

The reason endometriosis is so painful is that it is an inflamma-tory condition. **Essential fatty acids (EFAs)** can counter this by producing substances called prostaglandins which have a natural anti-inflammatory action. The best source of the omega fatty acids, which the body cannot make but has to get from the diet, is an unpolluted fish oil or, if your child is vegetarian, flaxseed oil. Aim to give her the equivalent of 1g a day. Many sufferers also have low levels of **zinc,** which has a potent anti-inflammatory action too. Compensate for this by supplementing the diet with at least 15mg a day.

Sufferers should cut out caffeine, chocolate and alcohol, which are all stimulants that can exacerbate this condition, and take a good **multivitamin** to provide **magnesium** which helps relax both the uterus and muscular tissue. The **B vitamins** are important too since they help generate the liver enzymes that can convert oestrogen in the form of oestradiol – which causes the endometrial cells to proliferate – into a safer form called oestriol which can be excreted. These all work best when taken together so invest in a good **vitamin B complex** supplement.

DL-phenylalanine (DLPA) is another natural painkiller which you can buy in your local health store. It works in 60 per cent of those who take it but takes several weeks to kick in. If there is no improvement after three weeks, it is not the solution. When it does work, the theory is that it promotes the production of endorphins – the body's own natural painkillers – and interferes with the brain's perception of pain by altering the action of the neurotransmitters or chemical messengers. Mail-order DLPA from Revital (0800 252875): 30 × 1000mg capsules cost £13.45. This formula includes vitamin B6 for better absorption, but do not use it for anyone who may be pregnant, breastfeeding, taking antidepressants or suffering from high blood pressure.

Saw palmetto, which is more traditionally used to support the prostate gland in men, can block the action of the sex hormone called follicle stimulating hormone (FSH), which is known to increase endometrial tissue. However, with a condition this serious, do not try to DIY treat at home. Instead, find a practitioner who has treated it successfully before and find a local support group.

Flower power Australian bush remedy combo: She Oak and Turkey Bush. A powerful combination to support and rebalance the female hormones.

Eye Problems

What's happening?

Probably the most common eye infection is **conjunctivitis**, or pinkeye, which is caused by a bacterial or viral infection of the conjunctiva – the transparent membrane that covers and protects the whites of the eyes and the inner eyelids. It is highly contagious and spreads via the yellow pussy discharge that will cause discomfort and which can 'glue' the eye shut during sleep. This also means there is a high risk of the infection spreading from one eye to the other. Allergic conjunctivitis is a reaction to pollen and so is seasonal but this condition, which can last up to seven days, can also follow an injury to the eye or exposure to a very smoky atmosphere.

A **stye** is a bacterial infection on the edge of the eyelid in one of the oil-secreting glands. It is usually caused by the staphylococcus bacterium and should pass within three days.

What to do

Even if just one eye has turned red from conjunctivitis, you will need to treat both. Start with a homemade herbal eyewash made up of **eyebright, goldenseal** and **raspberry leaf.** To make the wash, steep ½ teaspoon of each herb in a pint of hot water. Cool, strain and use. These three herbs have antibacterial and antiviral properties and also work to support the immune system to prevent infections. Goldenseal is bright yellow and will stain fingers and worktops so use with care. You can use this mix as an eyewash to bathe both eyes or use a dropper bottle to place a few drops into each eye. Repeat this treatment several times a day.

The homeopathic remedy for itchy, infected eyes is **Euphrasia,** which is made from eyebright. Give one dose of 12x or 6c potency pills three times a day for two days. If there is a thick, yellow discharge which glues the eyes shut after sleep, give **Pulsatilla** 12x or 6c, three times a day for two days. Mail-order homeopathic medicines from Ainsworths (020 7935 5330).

For a stye, do not attempt to squeeze or puncture the lesion, which will worsen the infection. Instead, bathe the eye as above and give **zinc** (see page 86) to support the immune system and one age-appropriate dose of a **betacarotene** supplement each day. Recurring styes can be a sign of a vitamin A deficiency. The body can use betacarotenes to convert to this antioxidant nutrient, which is specific to the eyes and will help soothe and heal its mucous membranes.

Flower power Australian bush remedy combo: Sunshine Wattle and Bush Fuchsia. This combo helps 'clear' the vision in every sense, literally and spiritually.

Fever

What's happening?

Technically, a fever is any rise in body temperature of at least 1°F above the normal body temperature of 98.6°F (0.6°C above 37°C). In fact, a younger child's temperature can easily vary by as much as 1°C/2°F, depending on what they are doing and how they are feeling. Also, although in adults the higher the temperature the more serious the illness, this does not apply to kids. A child with a mild cold, for instance, may have a fever of 40°C/104°F, while one with pneumonia may have a fever of only 37.7°C/100°F. In newborns, those systems that regulate body temperature are very unsophisticated and so listlessness and a poor appetite can often be better indications of sickness than temperature fluctuations.

In older children, a fever is a common symptom of infection and sickness. It is one of the body's natural defence mechanisms – a rise in temperature enhances the ability of the immune system to seek out and destroy bacteria and viruses – and a naturopath will tell you that if your child has a fever, this is an excellent sign that the body is working the way it is supposed to. A fever works to inhibit the reproduction of the bacteria and viruses that are causing the sickness and also helps the body flush out the resulting waste products and toxins.

In newborns and children under three, a very high fever can cause febrile seizures. This is very frightening but also very rare. If you suspect your child is having any kind of seizure, don't waste time. Call the doctor immediately or take them to the nearest A&E department.

What to do

Many natural healers will tell you to let a fever run its course but one advantage in bringing the fever down is that you can then work out what is going on underneath. If, for instance, the fever is a reaction to a cold, your child will soon look and feel much better. If there is a more serious infection, then bringing the body temperature down will make little or no difference. If tackling a fever of 38.3°C/101°F or lower, use warm fluids such as **chamomile tea** to encourage more sweating and take the naturo-pathic approach by letting the body do its own healing work.

If the fever rises above 38.3°C/101°F, you can use herbs to cool the body and promote further sweating. **Hyssop** is the best choice if your child is coughing and spluttering too. Add **yarrow** to a warm bath to prevent the fever from rising. **Blessed thistle** (*Cnicus benedictus*) is also traditionally used to reduce fever in childhood diseases, including measles and chicken pox. Mail-order supplies from Herbs of Grace on 01638 750140 and use as directed. If the temperature rises above 39.4°C/103°F, take your child to the doctor.

A fever increases the metabolic rate, making dehydration a risk. Keep your child hydrated with **organic fruit juices**, homemade **frozen fruit popsicles** and **broth-style soups**. Most kids will not want to eat when they feel this sick and keeping fluids in the body is more important than forcing food into them.

You can also help lower the body temperature or sweat out a fever by giving your child a massage using essential oils but remember to dilute them in a carrier oil first (see page 119). To cool the body use **peppermint** or **eucalyptus**. To promote sweat-ing, use **lavender, tea tree** or **yarrow**.

Flower power Australian bush remedy combo: Mountain Devil and Mulla Mulla will both help to bring down the fever.

Hay Fever

What's happening?

Hay fever – or allergic rhinitis – is a reaction of the mucous membranes of the eyes, nose and airways to seasonal pollens and other everyday allergens, including dust, feathers, animal hairs and environmental pollutants. When this happens, the body releases large numbers of antibodies to fight the perceived allergen but these antibodies also produce histamine which causes swelling and irritation to the body's own tissues.

Hay fever is rare in the under fives but very common in teens, especially where there is a family history of allergic reactions and related conditions such as asthma and eczema. If this is the case, you need to work at rebuilding and stabilizing the immune system.

What to do

Vitamin C not only supports the immune system, but helps the body defend itself against the consequences of having too much histamine released. It can also help reduce the release of histamine. In a study by scientists at the Arizona State University, researchers gave allergy sufferers, including patients with hay fever, increasing doses of vitamin C, starting with 500mg daily and increasing to 2000mg per day over a period of six weeks. They found that by the time the higher levels of vitamin C were reached, volunteers' histamine levels had dropped by 40 per cent.

Bioflavonoids are the substances that give fruits and vegetables their rich colours. They are synergistic with vitamin C which means if you use the two together, you will get even more health benefits. The best bioflavonoid for hay fever is **quercetin** which helps stabilize the cell membranes of those cells that would otherwise discharge their supply of histamine into the surrounding blood and tissue. A natural antihistamine, it will also work in the body to relieve any inflammation of the nasal passages, the bronchial airways and the throat. It is found naturally in red and yellow onions, shallots, squash, courgettes and broccoli (see Rainbow Foods, page 196) but it would be difficult to eat enough of these foods to get the full benefits.

Teens may turn their noses up at the notion of a nettle tea but the humble **stinging nettle** (*Urtica dioica*) is a hotbed of herbal pharmacological activity and one of the most effective natural remedies for hay fever. It contains both vitamins C and K, as well as immune-boosting proteins and an anti-inflammatory agent called **scopoletin**, which will counter the action of the body's histamine discharge.

*****

Five-star Tip

Country Life's Aller-Max formulation includes stinging nettles, bromelain, quercetin, vitamin C, grapeseed extract and vitamin A. The latter works to maintain the membrane surfaces of the body. 50 capsules cost £11.95. If you cannot find this at your local health store, mail-order from the Nutri Centre (020 7636 0422) or Revital (0800 252875) health stores.

A strong immune system will help protect from allergic reactions, including hay fever, and **echinacea** will support your child's natural defences.

If you know you have a hay fever sufferer in the family, a daily teaspoon of **local honey** dissolved in warm water should also help keep the symptoms at bay. Naturopaths say this works because it delivers a tiny dose of local pollen, which is usually the main trigger for an attack. This minuscule daily dose then helps the body build resistance so that when spring or summer arrives, and pollen is everywhere, the body is already protected.

Flower power Australian bush remedy combo: Fringed Violet and Dagger Hakea. Both remedies work to strengthen the body from the inside.

Headaches

What's happening?

Headaches are usually a sign of another problem. They may be linked, for example, to infection, to a cold or constipation, to a food allergy or intolerance (see page 169) and, of course, to emotional upsets such as exam nerves, fear and anxiety. Measles, flu and meningitis can cause headaches too, so can tension and stress. Headaches, especially migraines, which are more common where there is a family history of the condition, can also be a sign of changes to the blood vessels in the head.

If your child is crying and holding his or her head, then the underlying cause is likely to be more serious than nervous tension or an emotional upset. Rule out meningitis (by reading pages 28–33), and if in any doubt, call the doctor or take your child to hospital.

What to do

If your child has a headache that is accompanied by high fever, severe vomiting, a stiff neck, confusion, disorientation and extreme tiredness, see your doctor right away. If headaches are frequent and chronic, see the doctor too.

Conventional painkillers work best at the start and not halfway through a headache, and if you must give something like Ibuprofen, give it with food to avoid stomach upset. **Boswellia** is a herb that is just as powerful. Use the supplement made by Solgar. If you want to stick with the more natural treatments, start with a warm **peppermint tea** that can help relieve any congestion in the head. **Chamomile tea** is very calming and can help soothe a tension headache but most kids don't like the taste so you may get better results if you use a tincture and hide it in fruit juice.

Fried, greasy and extra fatty foods can all cause headaches, as can overeating, so serve light and nutritious snacks and meals (see Snack Attack and Rainbow Recipes, pages 165 and 213) until your child feels well again. Check food and drink labels and avoid foods that contain the flavouring agent monosodium glutamate (MSG), which can produce pounding headaches and what has become known as Chinese Restaurant Syndrome (see Additives, page 34).

Low blood sugar levels will also cause headaches. Prevent this by giving your kids foods that rank low (under 50) on the **Glycaemic Index** (GI) in order to maintain a more even release of energy throughout the day. Avoid sugary junk foods that will give an immediate energy hit and high followed by an equally rapid slump, which will make any headache worse. For an up-to-date list of GI food rankings, see page 179.

If you suspect the headache is linked to constipation, give **Solgar's ABC Dophilus powder**, a probiotic that will help re-regulate the digestive tract, and see Constipation, page 314.

Mi-Gon is formulated for migraines but works just as well with other headaches. An aromatherapy roll-on stick, it contains **sweet basil** and **peppermint oils**, both of which are analgesics, which means they relieve pain. Peppermint also has a cooling action on the skin. Simply roll Mi-Gon on the temples, about an inch above and between the eyes, and at the soft pulse points behind the ear lobes. The relief, when it works, should be instant. If nothing happens after fifteen minutes, it's not going to work so give up. (Mi-Gon costs £9.50 which includes p&p. To order, call 01526 832491.)

If Mi-Gon doesn't work, use **Migravoid,** made from the anti-inflammatory herb **butterbur**. Studies in adults show that using 50mg of standardized herb extract twice daily for 4–6 months can reduce migraine attacks by 62 per cent. Migravoid costs £24.95 for 50 capsules. Mail-order from Victoria Health on 0800 413596 and give an age-related dose.

Flower power Australian bush remedy combo: Emergency Essence, Five Corners, Paw Paw and Sturt Desert Rose. Emergency Essence relieves pain. Five Corners promotes self-confidence, Paw Paw supports the body through internal struggles, including headaches, and Sturt Desert Rose is for those who bottle up feelings and rarely cry.

Headlice

What's happening?

If you spot a tiny grey-white creature, just one eighth of an inch long (about 3 or 4mm) and with six little legs, in your child's hair, you need to get the whole family nit-busting. Headlice live only on humans, setting up camp on or close to the scalp where they can bite and suck up blood. They can be hard to spot so outwit them by using a torch. Look carefully at the hairline at the back of the neck where the females lay their eggs, which we call nits.

These will look like little white specks which you won't be able to brush out. It takes around eight days for nits to hatch into the adult headlice which can then live for up to five weeks. The females lay four or five eggs a day and will carry on until you stop them! The first tell-tale sign of an infection is usually a child absentmindedly scratching his or her head. This can create sores which, if left untreated, may become infected.

What to do

If you have a child under the age of ten, check for nits every night. It is much easier to prevent infestation at the outset than to break the life cycle and get rid of them for good once the lice have set up home. First check the base of the hairline for the eggs. Then use a metal comb to remove any adult lice and their eggs. (The plastic combs may be cheaper but the teeth usually spread which defeats the object.)

Stewart Distribution (01273 703461) sell an excellent **Tea Tree and Quassia Shampoo** and **Conditioner** that will get rid of head-lice for good. (Quassia is an infusion of woodchip and a natural insect repellent; tea tree is a powerful herbal disinfectant that will help prevent reinfection.) The shampoo is £7.95 for 250ml but to prevent infection you will need to use it only once a week. The conditioner, which costs £7.95 for 100ml, can be massaged into the scalp and onto dry hair each day to keep headlice away. You can also order a good quality metal comb, which costs £3.25. The new **Boots Alternatives** range also includes a good tea tree and lavender treatment, a leave-in conditioner and a fine-toothed comb.

The adult lice can survive for a day or so away from the body. They will be hiding in pillows, bedlinen, towels and clothes, so wash and change these regularly.

Flower power Australian bush remedy combo: Red Grevillea and Black-eyed Susan. These remedies will prevent itching and help the body cope with the stress of an infestation.

Impetigo

What's happening?

Impetigo is a highly infectious skin disorder caused by the staphylococcus or streptococcus bacteria and usually found around the lips, chin, nose and ears. Characterized by small and fragile pus-filled blisters, once these break open, it leaves infectious and weepy sores which will eventually dry to form a crusted scab. More common in kids than adults, impetigo can follow an injury such as sunburn or an insect bite, which causes a break in the skin allowing the infection to take hold.

The conventional treatment is antibiotics but natural remedies can be just as effective, especially if you adopt a comprehensive programme designed to support not only the immune system but the digestive and lymphatic systems, as well as your child's emotional frame of mind.

Poor hygiene does not cause this condition – it is the fluid in the blisters that transmits the disease. That said, it is helpful to keep the skin clean. Impetigo is so contagious it can be passed on via clothing so, during an infection, discreetly keep your child's towels, bedlinen, face cloths and clothing separate.

If you suspect an impetigo infection in an infant, especially a newborn, contact your doctor immediately.

What to do

In older kids, bring the infection under control by bathing the affected areas in a dilution of **tea tree oil** (dilute ten drops in a cup of warm water) several times a day. Use the superstrength **Desert Essence** brand which is eco-harvested, 100 per cent organic and as pure as you can get. Pat dry with a paper towel, which you must then discard.

Supplementing the diet with **essential fatty acids** (EFAs) will also help. These work to support the adrenal glands which sit atop the kidneys and which produce hormones to help fight infection and reduce inflammation. Oily fish are a good source of EFAs; if you want an alternative source, use **flaxseed** or **evening primrose oils**. The **B vitamins** are known as nature's own stress-busters so use a good quality multisupplement and **B complex** to supply these. **Vitamin A,** which maintains healthy skin, can also help fight this infection. For age-related doses, see page 64.

Vitamin C has anti-inflammatory and antibacterial properties. Take advantage of its natural synergy with the bioflavonoid **quercetin**, which will also reduce inflammation, and give these two nutrients combined. **Activated Quercetin** made by Natural Source combines quercetin with vitamin C. It costs £12.99 for 50 capsules. If not available at your local health store, mail-order from Revital (0800 252875). **Zinc** will also boost the immune system so, again, give an age-appropriate daily dose (see page 86).

The over-the-counter homeopathic remedy for impetigo is **Aurum 30**. For the best long-term results and to help prevent re-infection, consult a qualified homeopath who can prescribe a tailor-made regimen that will include a constitutional remedy factoring in your child's personality as well as medical history.

Try to discourage scratching at the sores, which will spread the infection. Use mittens – especially at night – with very young children who cannot resist temptation or don't understand why they must not scratch.

Flower power Australian bush remedy combo: **Black-eyed Susan** for stress and immune support, **Mountain Devil** and **Dagger Hakea** for psychological support.

Insomnia and Sleepnessness

What's happening?

Nobody's getting any sleep, that's what. Most children need ten to twelve hours' sleep a night – newborns sleep around sixteen hours a day – and if a child doesn't get the sleep he or she needs, you will pay for it with an irritable and fractious mood the following day. To tackle the problem, you need first to pinpoint the underlying cause, which can be as varied as emotional upset, an allergic reaction, stomach ache, or nasal congestion. In other words, lots of different things can affect the sleep pattern. Your child may have trouble getting off to sleep in the first place or may be waking at intervals throughout the night.

What to do

It goes without saying (almost) that you need to avoid giving your children any of the dietary stimulants that will keep them awake at night. These include any foods or drinks that contain caffeine, refined sugars or chocolate. Foods that will help a child to sleep include bananas, fish, dates, milk and turkey, all of which are rich in **tryptophan**. This is an animo acid which is crucial for the production of serotonin, the brain chemical that helps control mood and sleep. Researchers have found, for example, that adults who find it hard to get off to sleep are usually deficient in serotonin, the synthesis of which also requires large amounts of **vitamin B6** (pyridoxine, see page 70), which is found in carrots, cheese, avocado, fish, lentils, peas, potato, spinach, sunflower seeds and wholemeal flour. It is also present in milk, which is why a bedtime drink of **warm milk** can help. So will a warm **lavender** bath. (Use a lavender bath milk for very young children (see page 120).)

The B vitamins help calm the nervous system and one of the best sources for children over the age of twelve is **brewer's yeast**, which is high in these and other vitamins and minerals. Give a teaspoon at bedtime.

Since children respond so well to homeopathic remedies, either consult a qualified practitioner who can make a constitutional diagnosis or, if you prefer an over-the-counter remedy, use **Coffea cruda** (homeopathic coffee), which can help relieve both the nerves and the excitement that may be interfering with normal sleep patterns. This may sound unlikely but remember the basic tenet with homeopathy is that 'like cures like'.

Passion flower tincture can help in acute cases of insomnia and is excellent if you are travelling long-haul with a younger child, in which case you need to look for an alcohol-free version. If you can't find one locally, contact Revital (0800 252875).

You can help set the right mood in the bedroom by burning

relaxing oils such as **lavender, rose, sandalwood, chamomile** or **ylang ylang**. I use a plug-in, slow-release electric **vaporizer** (which can also work as a humidifier) in my daughter's bedroom when she can't sleep. Made by the essential-oil specialists Tisserand, it cost £17.99. Ask your local health store for details.

Calcium is a powerful sleep inducer but if you give a supplement you need to balance it by giving **magnesium** too. The ratio is 2:1 in favour of the calcium. To help re-establish good sleep patterns, give children over four years old 250mg of calcium and 125mg of magnesium in the morning and again at bedtime. Continue for several months or until the insomnia has passed.

Flower power Australian bush remedy combo: Black-eyed Susan, Crowea and Boronia. Black-eyed Susan supports the body through times of stress, Crowea promotes inner balance and Boronia will stop a racing mind.

Jealousy

What's happening?

It may be the arrival of a new baby or, worse, a new boyfriend in your life which has prompted outbursts of jealous tantrums or extra clingy behaviour. Whatever the trigger, the problem is insecurity, and this is one of those times when **flower remedies** really come into their own.

What to do

The flower remedies I like best are the Australian bush remedies. They are so contemporary, and not only address common emotional problems such as jealousy, but pinpoint everyday problems in the modern family such as lack of communication, long-held resentments and sibling rivalry.

If you prefer to stick to the longer-established English flower remedies in the Bach flower range, you will need to use **Holly**. And if jealous behaviour follows a divorce or separation, then combine it with **Pine** since this is the remedy for guilt and most kids blame themselves when a family breaks up.

To make your own combinations, mix two drops from each of the remedies you have selected in an empty 30ml dropper bottle which you can buy from the chemist. Top this mixture up with still mineral water and give four drops of the mixture, four times a day, until the problem passes. The Bach flower remedies cost £3.15 each for 10ml. You can mail order all the individual remedies, plus the world-famous **Rescue Remedy**, from Nelson's on 020 7495 2404.

Flower power Australian bush remedy: Bush Gardenia. This is *the* Australian bush remedy for jealousy. The Latin name *Gardenia megasperma* means Big Seed and this is the remedy you need to use to strengthen family bonds, not only between brothers and sisters but between generations. (Keep it on hand for Christmas!) It is also useful for teens who may be going off the rails due to drug or other addiction problems, and who may be feeling that everyone else in the family is too busy getting on with their own lives to even notice. Bush Gardenia will improve communication between parents and kids and promote a more loving relationship between younger siblings. (To find out how to take these remedies for best effect, see page 124.)

Lactose Intolerance

What's happening?

Lactose intolerance is the inability to digest the milk sugar lactose. It is not the same as a milk allergy – where the milk can be digested but then causes problems with the immune system – but is due to a deficiency in the enzyme **lactase** which is manufactured in the small intestine, where it splits lactose into glucose and galactose. The symptoms, which usually start up to two hours after the consumption of dairy foods, include gas, diarrhoea and stomach cramping, and are the result of undigested lactose fermenting in the colon. For most adults with this condition it is just a fact of life, but it is much more problematic (and uncommon) in infants and children, where it may be the result of a previous gastrointestinal disorder that has damaged the lining of the gut and where, if left unchecked, it can cause vomiting and delay development and weight gain.

What to do

Thankfully, you can use supplements not only to replenish lactase levels but also to build up the population of the good gut bacteria that aid digestion. Lots of adults now take these replacement bacteria, or **probiotics**, which were first used in agriculture to improve growth and yield, but few parents realize that children, especially those who have been bottle-fed or given antibiotics, will benefit too. For infants, use **Biocare's Bifidobacterium Infantis powder**, which costs £22.50 (mail-order on 0121 433 3727); for children over two use **Solgar's ABC Dophilus powder**, which costs £13.85 for 49.6g and is for up to four years of age. For local stockists, call 01442 890355. Older kids will benefit from **Nutrition Now's Lacto Safe**, which works naturally to help the body digest milk and dairy foods. Mail-order from Victoria Health on 0800 413596.

Flower power Australian bush remedy: Paw paw is the bush remedy for all internal struggles, including digestive problems.

Measles

What's happening?

This is a viral infection which passes from one child to another via air or droplets from sneezing or coughing. It has a long incubation period – ten to twelve days – and is contagious from around day five of this period. Of course, most parents don't know their child has measles until the first rash appears, by which time the virus will probably have passed to every other child in the family (and any that have visited too). The first signs are usually a runny nose, conjunctivitis, fever and a cough. You may see white spots on the inside lining of the cheek, which will soon be followed by the all-too-familiar red rash, which first appears behind the ears, under the arms and on the face and neck. As more and more spots appear, they start to merge to form red patches over the whole body. This rash will last for five to seven days. Kids with measles may also throw up, have diarrhoea and complain of abdominal pain. But once the fever – which can climb to as high as 40.5°C/105°F – breaks, the patient will start to feel better. The other bit of good news, if you want to look on the bright side, is that once a child has had measles, the body builds a life-long immunity and will never have this sickness again. This is why breastfeeding mothers pass the same immunity to their babies, who then remain protected for the first six months of life. Of course, measles is rare now because most parents still opt into the government's MMR vaccination programme which covers measles, mumps and rubella (German measles) and which then provides 'herd immunity' (see page 13). These jabs are usually given at fifteen months and just before school entry. For more on this, see page 5. German measles is one of the mildest contagious diseases of childhood but is highly dangerous to pregnant women since it can cause miscarriage or congenital abnormalities of the foetus.

The reason measles is serious is because it can cause complications, including pneumonia, and encephalitis which is an inflammation of the lining of the brain. If the fever tops 40.5°C/105°F, if your child has a seizure or if you suspect any of the above, get immediate medical attention.

What to do

Vitamin A is important for skin healing so give your child an age-appropriate daily dose (see page 66) and carry on for a fortnight. **Vitamin C**, combined with **bioflavonoids**, is a powerful immune booster. I like **Biocare's Vitamin C and Bilberry** (call 0121 433 3727).

To clear any eye infection (usually conjunctivitis) see page 334. The **medicinal mushrooms** from Asia will also help rebuild resistance to bacterial and viral diseases. Give an age-related dose of **Triton**, which combines shiitake, reishi and cordyceps mushrooms. Triton costs £13.50 for 60 × 500mg tablets and is available by mail order on 01273 625988.

Chamomile not only helps reduce a fever but stimulates the immune system too. Make soothing popsicles by brewing and then freezing chamomile tea, or use a ready-made tincture. Good herbal suppliers include Bioforce (01294 27734), Biohealth (01634 290115), Napiers (0131 343 6638) and Herbs of Grace (01638 750140).

Keep your child hydrated with fluids and give a soothing oatmeal bath to relieve itching. Fill a small linen or muslin bag with the grain to pop into the bath. Add a few drops of lavender oil or a tablespoon of lavender bath milk (see page 120) to make the whole experience more relaxing.

Flower power Australian bush remedy combo: To help bring down the fever, give **Mountain Devil** and **Mulla Mulla**.

Mumps

What's happening?

Mumps is a viral infection which targets and affects the salivary glands, especially the partoid glands next to the ear. It is spread via saliva and has an incubation period of fourteen to twenty-one days. The first signs of an infection include a fever, headache, no appetite, aching muscles and chills. The following day, your child will complain of a pain in the ear and under the jaw. For the next few days, the salivary glands start to swell, making talking, eating and swallowing uncomfortable and painful. From this point, your child will remain infectious until about the ninth day. That said, most UK children are now vaccinated against mumps as part of the controversial MMR vaccine (see page 5). Mumps, which is most common in five- to fifteen-year-olds, usually runs its own course. It is less contagious than either measles or chicken pox and complications are rare. One of the worst happens when the virus attacks the testicles in males, causing short-term pain and swelling and a risk of long-term infertility in teens and younger adults.

What to do

A child with mumps needs to be isolated until the swollen glands return to normal size. They need **plenty of rest** and **plenty of water and other healthy drinks** – herbal teas, diluted organic fruit juices or healing herbal popsicles – to replace those fluids lost during the initial fever. Apply warm or cool compresses (see page 107) to the swollen glands to ease the pain and **eliminate unhealthy saturated fats from the diet,** which can be difficult to digest at the best of times and even more difficult when the body is coping with infection. Swallowing will be painful and acidic foods, such as tomatoes or orange juice, all exacerbate the problem. **Avoid other citrus fruits** too.

For kids over twelve, use **shiitake mushrooms** to boost the immune system and accelerate recovery (see page 111). For younger children, use **echinacea** (either in tincture or chewable tablet form), and give an age-appropriate dose (see page 101). **Zinc** also kick-starts the immune response. Use a formulation such as **Nutrition Now's Rhino Zinc** made for children, and give the equivalent of 10mg a day for 10 days.

At the onset of infection, warm **chamomile tea** will not only soothe your child and help him or her sleep but will assist in bringing down the fever too. If your child hates the taste, brew the tea and freeze it overnight in homemade lollipop moulds to make a healing herbal popsicle.

Homeopaths report excellent results with this and other common childhood viral infections. For the best results, consult a qualified practitioner who has extensive clinical experience of working with children. The practitioner will make a constitutional diagnosis which will take into account your child's personality and preferences, as well as previous medical history. If you want to use over-the-counter remedies, give **Belladonna 30x or 9c** to a child whose right-side gland is more swollen than the left, who has a high fever and whose face is flushed. If the pain has reached the ears, give the patient **Phytolacca 12x** or **6c**, and if the left gland is more swollen than the right, give **Rhus toxico-dendron 30x** or **9c**. If the testicles are affected, give **Mercurius solubilis 12x** or **6c**.

Flower power Australian bush remedy combo: Peach-flowered **Tea Tree** to rid the body of infection, and **Hibbertia** to regulate and rebalance the partoid glands.

Nappy Rash

What's happening?

Nappy rash is an inflammation of the skin, usually in response to the chemicals and enzymes in excreted urine and faeces, and exacerbated by the build-up of heat in a soiled nappy which traps this noxious mix against your poor baby's bottom. That said, there are two different types of nappy rash – one caused by this contact, the other by a fungal infection of candida albicans, which is present in the digestive tract. A contact rash usually looks red, swollen and irritated, or the skin may be dry and scaling. With a fungal infection, the baby's bottom will be shiny and red. If you're not able to distinguish between these two, ask your health visitor or doctor to tell you which type of rash you are dealing with. Most common at around nine months, nappy rash can occur at any stage that a child is still in nappies. It can appear after a dose of antibiotics or a bout of stomach upset and diarrhoea. In more extreme cases, an impetigo infection can also follow (see page 344).

What to do

If you take the right steps, you should be able to clear this problem in two or three days. Disposable nappies are always more likely to trigger nappy rash than cotton ones so if you can face switching until the problem is resolved then do so.

Keep the baby's bottom scrupulously clean with regular nappy changes and bathe the whole bottom with one of the disinfecting and soothing **floral waters** that are safe to use with infants. Floral waters have the same properties as essential oils but do not need diluting and have a more gentle action. Keep a selection – especially **lavender** and **calendula** – of the high quality organic oils supplied by Natural Health Remedies (NHR). Contact this company on 020 8746 0890 or visit the website at www.nhr.kz.

Nappy rash can be a reaction to certain foods the mother is eating, especially yeasted breads, citrus fruits, sugar, caffeine and dairy products. Breastfeeding mothers can literally dilute this effect by drinking plenty of filtered water.

If you suspect a candida infection, give your baby a **probiotic** supplement in powder form. Biocare's **Bifidobacterium Infantis** costs £22.50 for 60g. Mail-order direct from the company on 0121 433 3727. For babies up to one year old, give a quarter of a teaspoon mixed with a little warm filtered water.

Treat a red and irritated bottom with **calendula cream** and **powder**. Weleda's Calendula Baby Powder costs £2.40 for 75g and is designed to beat nappy rash. The treatment cream is £4.20 for 75ml. To order, call 0115 944 8222. For more information on this range, which includes a calendula barrier cream, visit the website at www.weleda.co.uk. **Evening primrose oil** is also an excellent natural anti-inflammatory agent, as is a **vitamin E cream**.

To prevent further infection, expose your baby's bottom to fresh air and sunlight where you can. If using cotton nappies, make sure they are cleaned with mild and natural detergent such as calendula soap to avoid further chemicals coming into contact with the skin.

Flower power Australian bush remedy: Spinifex promotes internal cleansing.

Nosebleeds

What's happening?

Nosebleeds are caused by a rupture of the small blood vessels of the septum, the fleshy middle partition of the nose. Unless a nosebleed follows a blow to the head – in which case see the doctor – there is no need to panic. The damage can be a result of too-vigorous nose-blowing, antisocial nose-picking, sneezing or coughing, or an emotional response. The most awe-inspiring nosebleed I ever saw happened when my dad walked into the bedroom I shared with my teenage sisters to tell us Elvis Presley had died. One of my sister's friends – a teenage fan of the King – was doing what the kids now would call a sleepover. She sat bolt upright, burst into hysterical sobs and shocked us all by soaking the pillow with the blood from the nosebleed that ensued.

What to do

The trick to stopping a nosebleed is to get the blood to clot. To do this, **sit the patient in an upright position, tip the head back, ask him or her to keep the mouth open and, with your thumb and fingers, apply pressure to the lower half of the nose.** Imagine you are squeezing each side of the septum. If you can both hold this position for ten minutes, you have a better chance of success than if you give up after just three or four. If after twenty minutes the bleeding hasn't stopped, call the doctor's surgery.

If your child is suffering from frequent nosebleeds, you need to strengthen the tiny blood vessels that are rupturing all too easily. The two most important bioflavonoids that help do this are **rutin** and **bilberry**. Both work even better when combined with **vitamin C**. One of the better products you can use is **Biocare's Children's Vitamin C and Bilberry**. Mail-order on 0121 433 3727 and give one capsule to kids aged five and older. To adjust this dose for toddlers, see page 65. **Vitamin K** supports the blood-clotting mechanism and so is useful for children with a recurring problem. Give 15mcg (micrograms, not milligrams) twice a day for a month and monitor any improvements.

Nettle tea, which is a hotbed of pharmacological activity, contains **vitamins A and C** which both work to strengthen the mucous membrane of the septum. Even better, it provides an easy-to-absorb form of **iron**. Unfortunately, it has a strong planty taste which most kids will turn their noses up at. Get around this problem by combining it with sweeter-tasting orange or apple juice and freezing this mix to make fruit popsicles.

The over-the-counter homeopathic remedy for nosebleeds is **Ferrum phosphoricum 6x** or **6c**. Give the patient one little pill every ten minutes for up to four doses, until the bleeding stops.

Flower power Australian bush remedy: Illawarra Flame Tree. This works to support the body through minor setbacks.

Osgood-Schlatter Disease

What's happening?

Osgood-Schlatter disease or osteochondrosis may not be all that common but if it happens to your footballing or sports-mad sons or daughters, they're going to be devastated. Although described by doctors as a temporary condition, it can last as long as a year – try telling an eleven-year-old football-mad boy he can't do *any* sport for twelve months and see how popular that's going to make you.

What's happening, in simple terms, is that the bones of the leg are growing too fast for the tendons that attach muscle to bone to keep up. The problem will be exacerbated if your child is keen on sport, which can overstress the knee joint. You might be tempted to dismiss leg pains as normal growing pains but when your child complains specifically of sore knees, which then start to look swollen and painful, you will need a check-up to confirm the diagnosis. Osgood-Schlatter can affect boys and girls and is most common around puberty but very rare after the age of sixteen.

The doctor may prescribe aspirin or support tights, and in extreme cases a leg cast or splint may be used to take pressure off this part of the leg. But since what you are dealing with is an inflammatory condition there are some natural remedies that will help to bring down the inflammation and control the associated swelling and pain.

What to do

Two of the most powerful anti-inflammatory remedies you can use are **bromelain,** an enzyme derived from fresh pineapple juice, and **boswellia,** a herbal resin extracted from the gum of the Indian *Boswellia serrata* tree. Bromelain is available on its own but is also now starting to be incorporated into adult joint formulations. One of the best is LifeTime's **Advanced Joint Support** formula, a US supplement which also includes glucosamine, collagen, chondroitin and MSM. Available only from Victoria

Health (0800 413596), give an age-appropriate dosage (adults take three tablets a day, so give kids aged between eleven and fifteen one tablet daily) and try to persuade your child to switch to a non-weight-bearing form of sport, such as swimming, until the inflammation clears for good.

Nobody is making a supplement that combines both these anti-inflammatory agents so you will need to buy your boswellia separately. This is as effective in controlling muscular pain as Ibuprofen and other over-the-counter painkillers so treat it with respect and keep the bottle out of the reach of younger kids. **Solgar's Boswellia serrata** costs £14.75 for 60 veggie capsules. For local stockists, call 01442 890355. (Do not confuse *Boswellia serrata* with *Boswellia carteri*. Both are often called frankincense, but they have different actions in the body.)

Nutritional doctors recommend **vitamin E** (400 International Units a day) and **selenium** (50 micrograms, three times a day), but you will both need to be patient since it can take up to six weeks to see any results or improvement.

Flower power Australian bush remedy combo: Sturt Desert Rose and Emergency Essence, for general inflammation and pain.

Period Pains and PMT

What's happening?

To doctors, menstrual cramps are known as dysmenorrhoea, which means painful menstruation. This is one of the most common gynaecological complaints, with more than half of all females suffering at some time in their lives. A period can last from two to eight days. The cycle itself can range from nineteen to thirty-five days although the average is twenty-eight days.

What is happening during menstruation is that the rich lining of the womb, which the body had prepared to nurture a fertilized egg, is shed. A teen who is suffering from severe pain during menstruation needs to see the doctor to rule out underlying causes such as an ectopic pregnancy, endometriosis (see page 332), ovarian cysts, pelvic inflammatory disease or fibroids.

What to do

Females who suffer from cramping have been shown to produce greater levels of **prostaglandins** – the hormones secreted by the uterine lining – and this can be exacerbated by a diet that is rich in saturated fats from meat and dairy products. Many teens report massive relief when these foods, along with high sugar and highly processed foods, are eliminated from the diet. Period pains will be made worse by any underlying digestive disorder, especially constipation, so a **high-fibre diet** and a good quality **probiotic** will also help.

Evening primrose oil is rich in **gammalinoleic acid** (GLA), an anti-inflammatory prostaglandin that can counter the inflammatory hormones causing pain. Your daughter should take a supplement providing the equivalent of 250mg of GLA a day for three months and monitor the relief.

Nutritionists recommend **niacin** (vitamin B3, see page 68), which triggers a dilation of the blood vessels to improve blood flow to the contracting uterus. Give your daughter 50–100mg every day for five days only, starting with the first period pains. Niacin can cause flushing so look for a non-flushing form. (If flushing does occur, do not panic. It will pass after about ten minutes.) **Vitamin B6** (see page 70) is important too. All the B vitamins work best when taken together so invest in a good **vitamin B complex**. A medium-sized banana provides a quarter of the amount of the daily dose of vitamin B6 most girls and women need. Remember, though, the contraceptive pill increases the body's demand for this nutrient.

Underlying blood sugar imbalances are exacerbated by premenstrual tension and will be made worse by yo-yo dieting and junk foods. To maintain even blood sugar levels, persuade your daughter to eat foods from the lower ranks of the **GI Index** (see page 179), particularly during menstruation.

Hidden candida (yeast) infections are also highly implicated in PMT and period pains and may be a root cause if your daughter has taken antibiotics in the past. To tackle this infection, see page 387.

A qualified herbalist can tailor-make a regimen to help rebalance hormones. To find one in your area, contact the **British Naturopathic Association** on 01458 840072, which holds a list of qualified naturopaths who combine herbalism with nutrition and homeopathy in their treatment programmes. The **National Institute of Medical Herbalists** is on 01392 426022. The **British Herbal Medicine Association** is on 01453 751389.

Moderate exercise – anathema to most teenage girls who'd rather stay slim by starving themselves – will encourage the liver to metabolize excess hormones and flush them out of the body, and lead to a gradual improvement every month. **Yoga**, which also works to balance the endocrine system, is now so fashionable that your teen may be persuaded to take it up. For details, see page 148.

If you are looking for organic tampons and sanitary towels, the **Natracare range** from Bodywise is certified GM-free. Unlike commercial products that have been bleached whiter than white using chlorine, the Natracare range, which uses 100 per cent organic cotton, contains no chemicals, binding ingredients, surfactants, additives or synthetic materials such as rayon. Contact Bodywise on 01275 371764.

Flower power Australian bush remedy combo: She Oak, Crowea and Peach-flowered Tea Tree. She Oak is the female remedy, Crowea will help rebalance hormones and Peach-flowered Tea Tree can prevent mood swings.

Polycystic Ovary Syndrome (PCOS)

What's happening?

A hidden hormonal disorder believed to affect up to one in ten girls and women – some as young as sixteen – this condition can be difficult to diagnose, not least because in 50 per cent of cases there are no symptoms. In the other 50 per cent, signs of polycystic ovaries include sudden and unexplained weight gain, excess facial hair, adult acne and, in older women trying for a baby, fertility problems. It is the result of too much of the male hormone testosterone – remember, both sexes have both male and female hormones present, what counts is the balance between the two. PCOS sufferers also have a problem controlling blood sugar levels.

With PCOS, the ovaries are covered with a string of tiny, fluid-filled cysts which make the excess testosterone. This hormone is usually carried in the bloodstream by a substance called sex hormone-binding globulin. Without it, there are 'free' testosterone molecules which then bind in the wrong places, including under the skin where they cause acne and excess facial hair.

This condition is inherited so if you have it, Mum, there's a good chance your daughter will have it too. The conventional treatment is a low-dose contraceptive pill which can help control the more obvious symptoms – including heavy periods and adult acne – but according to natural health practitioners and even some doctors themselves this treatment can make the condition worse.

What to do

One of the most common symptoms of PCOS is a tendency to put on weight, and when this happens, the amount of sex hormone-binding globulin, which is made by the liver and which would normally mop up excess testosterone, decreases. This is why **reducing body weight** is a crucial first step in managing the symptoms. Nobody can cure PCOS so the key to coping with it is to adopt a combination of **natural remedies** and **dietary changes** that will reduce symptoms. Start, for example, by persuading your teen to eat less carbohydrate in her diet and instead to eat smaller and more frequent high-protein meals.

Find a qualified herbalist, homeopath or naturopath in your area who has experience with this condition, and contact the nationwide support group, **Verity**, at pcos.org.uk.

Get a copy of Colette Harris's groundbreaking book on this long-ignored condition. Colette, a PCOS sufferer who is also the editor of *Here's Health* magazine, has done more in the UK to bring this condition out of the shadows than anyone else and her efforts should be supported, not least because new genetic research now shows how women with PCOS are seven times more likely to suffer from both cardiovascular problems and diabetes in later life. *PCOS – A Woman's Guide to dealing with Polycystic Ovary Syndrome* by Colette Harris with Dr Adam Carey (Thorsons, £9.99) includes details of the DIY natural health regimen Colette adopted, which, to the astonishment of doctors, cleared her ovaries of all cysts.

The **Centre for Nutritional Medicine** (020 7907 1660),

cofounded by Dr Carey, can test for PCOS. It costs £80 and all consultations at the centre include nutritional advice. A medically qualified herbalist will tailor-make a treatment plan that includes the hormone balancing (adaptogenic) herb **agnus castus**. Contact the **National Institute of Medical Herbalists** on 01392 426022. For online information and to exchange treatment tips with other PCOS sufferers and their families, visit www.pcosupport. org.

Flower power Australian bush remedy combo: She Oak, Turkey Bush and Crowea. These are the remedies that help re-balance the female hormones.

Psoriasis

What's happening?

The skin is not just a protective wrapping. It is the body's largest organ, and so the best place to tackle all skin complaints is from the inside out. That can mean changing the diet to avoid certain foods, such as the gluten in wheat which can exacerbate the problem, and taking even more care with the products being used to wash the skin and keep it clean.

Psoriasis is the result of a defect in the skin which causes cells to multiply 1,000 times faster than normal skin cells. These extra cells then pile up to cause the silvery scaling that is the hallmark of this condition. In 50 per cent of cases, the problem is inherited, and while there is no magic cure, there are lots of things that will help you manage the symptoms and, eventually, keep the skin clear.

One theory about the underlying cause of psoriasis is that the body cannot metabolize saturated fats from meat products properly. Sufferers have also been found to be lacking in both vitamin A and zinc.

What to do

Vitamin D can help but the body only makes this when exposed to natural light, especially sunshine, so try to make sure sufferers get outside into natural light for twenty minutes a day. This is also part of the treatment plan for those who make their way to the Dead Sea, where skin clinics report excellent results thanks to the combination of safe sunlight and mineral-rich waters.

To treat the outside of the skin, stick with a natural and non-abrasive product. I like the **Zambesia Botanica** range, which includes a gentle but effective scalp treatment. A traditional African remedy, which was discovered by an Englishman who had suffered from psoriasis for forty-five years until he used it, the active ingredient comes from the *Kigelia africana* tree. (Locals call it the 'sausage tree' since the fruit pods hang down from the branches looking just like sausages.) The Zambesia Botanica range includes creams and shampoos. The scalp formula costs £8.95 for 100ml. Mail-order from Farmacia (020 7404 8808).

Lots of sufferers also report great success with another herbal remedy called **Psoriaflora,** which contains *Mahonia aquifolium.* According to Canadian research, this plant contains an active ingredient which has been shown to help inhibit the abnormal skin growth rates that cause the condition. This cream, available from Victoria Health (0800 413596), can also relieve associated itching, scaling, redness and skin irritation.

Flower power Australian bush remedy combo: Little Flannel Flower and Billy Goat Plum. Little Flannel Flower is for children with a tendency to take on the troubles of the world; Billy Goat Plum is for all skin problems.

Scarlet Fever

What's happening?

The name may strike terror in the heart but all you are dealing with is a bacterial infection that is causing a sore throat and a tell-tale light pink or red rash of fine, raised spots that will feel like scratchy sandpaper when you touch it. There will be a headache, sore throat, fever and even vomiting before this rash appears, usually twelve hours to two days later, in the warmer parts of the body such as under the arms, behind the knees and in the groin area. It then spreads to the trunk and extremities. This rash will last up to seven days and then the affected skin will peel or flake off. Another sign of scarlet fever is a swollen red tongue.

What to do

Scarlet fever is always highly contagious. It is caused by virulent streptococcus bacteria which, if left unchecked, can trigger complications including, at its most extreme, rheumatic fever, an inflammatory disease that can damage the heart. If you suspect this infection, visit the doctor, who will confirm the diagnosis with a throat swab. Also consult a qualified natural health practitioner who can help you to support your child's body through treatment.

Herbal milk baths (see page 120) made from **lavender** or **calendula flowers** will help relieve irritability and tetchiness and promote lymphatic flow to help flush out the toxins generated by this infection.

Herbal lollipops or popsicles not only disguise herbal remedies but offer relief to a throat that can feel as if it's on fire. Either add a herbal tincture such as antibacterial **goldenseal** to a fruit juice and freeze, or make a soothing herbal tea from **chamomile** or **cleavers** and freeze the tea to make a soothing lolly to relieve the pain and numb the affected area. You can mail-order quality herbs from the Organic Herb Trading Company (01823 401104), Napiers (0131 343 6683) and Herbs of Grace (01638 750140).

Bacteria-fighting and immune-boosting **herbal throat lozenges** designed to soothe sore throats are now widely on sale in health stores. Blackmores (020 8842 3956) sell an excellent formula that combines **vitamin C, echinacea** and **eucalyptus**: 24 lozenges cost £4.15. Give one lozenge every hour until the acute phase has passed.

Naturopaths take the view that an acute disease like this is nature's way of ridding the body of a toxic infection, and argue that if you use aspirin or other allopathic drugs you send the infection deeper into the body. **Vitamin E** can help protect against this. Check page 76 for age-appropriate dosages. To make your own powerful herbal remedy for scarlet fever, combine equal parts of **echinacea** with **myrrh gum** and immune-supporting **capsicum** (cayenne). For convenience use ready-made tinctures. For suppliers and techniques, see Phytomedicine, pages 99–113.

Support immune function by cutting out sugar and dairy products until this infection has passed. Adopt a more nourishing diet with chicken broth and light vegetable soups. Your child is going to have a hard time swallowing so make it easier for him or her.

Flower power Australian bush remedy combo: Black-eyed Susan, Mountain Devil and Dagger Hakea. This combination supports the body through times of extra stress and infection and brings down a fever.

Sinusitis

What's happening?

The sinuses are, in effect, open spaces in the skull. They come in pairs and there are four sets of them: two spaces just behind the bridge of the nose, two in the upper nose, two in the forehead just above the eyebrow, and two under each eye just to the side of the nose. Their job is to warm, moisten and filter the air coming from outside into the lungs. The trouble with spaces in the body, however, is that they are the first places to become congested when any kind of infection takes hold.

When the sinuses are congested, blocked, irritated or inflamed, they can trigger a whole range of secondary symptoms including earache, headache, toothache, pain in the face, loss of the sense of smell, bad breath and tenderness in those affected areas. If you spot swelling or puffiness around the eyes, trouble is brewing so get to the doctor quick. Sinusitis, if it's not treated, can lead to meningitis or pneumonia so don't take any chances.

What to do

Chronic sinusitis is often linked to asthma and is the result of an allergic reaction. That means it won't go away until you identify the food or environmental triggers and remove them. Dairy products and milk are not helpful since they trigger the production of even more and thicker mucus which will be harder to drain so be strict and cut down on both. **Chicken broth** has the opposite effect: it will thin the mucus causing the congestion and speed up drainage so serve this for lunch every other day.

Betacarotenes convert to **vitamin A** in the body which can help heal inflamed mucous membranes. Give an age-related dosage of a betacarotene supplement once a day for five days. A low-dose **zinc lozenge** formulated for kids will also help boost the immune system to fight off secondary and further infection.

Start the day with a **homemade lemonade**, combining the juice of two lemons in hot water and organic maple syrup. This also helps relieve congestion by cutting mucus production.

Homeopathy is excellent for helping both the chronic and acute forms of this condition, but because it may be linked to asthma and other underlying allergies, your child will benefit more from a proper consultation than a DIY regimen. To find a qualified homeopath in your area, contact the Society of Homeopaths on 01604 621400. To find a doctor who is also a qualified homeopath, call the British Homeopathic Association (020 7935 2163).

If the doctor has prescribed antibiotics, which is the usual treatment for this condition, make sure you supplement the diet with a good quality **probiotic** which will rebuild levels of the good bacteria in the gut that help to keep us healthy but which get wiped out by antibiotics. Solgar's new **Advanced Acidophilus Plus** (60 veggie capsules cost £7.95) is OK for kids over four. For toddlers and infants, use the **ABC Dophilus powder** which costs £13.85 for 49.6g. For local stockists, call 01442 890355.

Flower power Australian bush remedy: Dagger Hakea helps relieve congestion.

Sore Throat

What's happening?

Pharyngitis is an inflammation of the throat; laryngitis is an inflammation of the voice box, and tonsilitis, as the name suggests, is an inflammation of the tonsils. What all three conditions have in common is that your child will present with a pretty nasty sore throat. Most sore throats are caused by either a viral or a bacterial infection. In children, a sore throat is usually accompanied by a head cold, a runny nose and an ear infection (see page 327), and while the majority of sore throats are minor infections which can be cleared at home, some are linked to more serious conditions such as scarlet fever (see page 367) which need immediate medical attention.

What to do

When dealing with a sore throat, the first thing you need to do is make an assessment of what type of infection it is. The most virulent of the infections causing sore throats is the streptococcus infection, which will spread through a family and playmates like wildfire. Streptococcus infections are more common in children aged three or over and the symptoms will be very sudden. One minute your child seems fine, the next it is obvious he or she is sick.

A streptococcus infection usually triggers a high fever with red and swollen tonsils. Look for white splotches on the tonsils and check the lymph nodes at the side of the throat, which will be tender and sore. A child with a strep infection will look and feel very sick. If you suspect this is the cause of the sore throat, take the child to the doctor.

If there is a history of scarlet or rheumatic fever, get the doctor to check every sore throat your child has. Otherwise, if you think you are dealing with a more common viral infection, which is usually accompanied by runny eyes, nose and a cough, give herbal lozenges made from **echinacea** and **vitamin C** and follow the advice given for soothing a sore throat with scarlet fever (page

367). Nature's Plus kids' **zinc lozenges** combine immune-boosting zinc with echinacea, olive leaf extract and ginger: 60 tablets cost £7.49. Mail-order from Revital (0800 252875).

Ginger is rich in manganese which helps build resistance to infection and disease. It also contains immune-boosting zinc and the anti-stress B vitamins. Make a ginger cordial or syrup (see page 194) or use a tincture. You can make a simple but soothing drink by combining lemon or lime juice with manuka honey, hot water and grated fresh ginger to help the body clear out the toxins from this infection. **Flaxseed oil**, which is rich in the **essential fatty acids** (EFAs), will also support a body that is fighting off and recovering from an infection.

Flower power Australian bush remedy combo: Bush Fuchsia, Bush Iris and Flannel Flower. Bush Fuchsia helps clear blockages, Bush Iris can soothe the pain and irritation and Flannel Flower boosts energy levels.

Stomach Cramps

What's happening?

Stomach ache and cramping is very common in kids. If these are the result of food poisoning, the onset will be sudden and dramatic and the body will try to 'throw out' the poison through vomiting and diarrhoea. Overeating is a common cause of stomach pains, as is constipation (see page 314, especially if your child has not had a bowel movement in the last 48 hours or is passing hard stools). Sometimes the reason is as simple as overexcitement, nervousness or anxiety, which is where the Australian flower remedy combo (see below) can quickly help redress the balance.

Stomach ache can also be a sign of an underlying urinary tract infection which you also need to investigate to rule out. Foul-smelling or cloudy urine is an obvious sign, although a low-grade infection may show no symptoms at all, making it more difficult to diagnose.

What to do

Avoid solid foods until the pain has gone. For older kids (aged eight upwards), try soothing **ginger** or **cinnamon teas** to help the gut settle back down again. If you think an infection is causing the cramping – if all the kids in class have had the same problem all weekend then common sense tells you this must be a bug – serve a homemade syrup (see page 194) and add antiviral and antibacterial **echinacea** tincture which will help boost the immune system too.

Soothe the stomach with the heat from a **warm water bottle** which your child can hold over his or her tummy, and burn relaxing **lavender** in an oil burner or vaporizer (see page 121). You can also dilute the oil in a carrier or base oil (such as almond) and massage it into the stomach to help relieve the tension there.

If you suspect a urinary infection may be the real culprit, make your own **lemon barley water** (see page 222). Persuade your child to drink three or four cups a day. Avoid fizzy drinks until the infection has passed.

Slippery elm heals and soothes the digestive tract, especially where there is inflammation resulting from infection. Make your own herbal medicine by mixing one teaspoon of the powdered herb in 600ml/1 pint of boiling water. Blend well, allow to cool and add antibacterial **cinnamon** to improve the flavour. Allow your child to drink this mix, which will coat and protect the lower colon, throughout the day and preferably on an empty stomach. Napier's herbalists (0131 343 6683) have a powder which costs £6.05 for 95g.

Flower power Australian bush remedy combo: Grey Spider Flower and Bottlebrush. Grey Spider Flower is the remedy for the sudden onset of sometimes frightening symptoms. Bottlebrush helps rebalance the digestive system.

Sunburn

What's happening?

Sunburn is usually a first degree burn where the skin turns red or pink as it becomes swollen and painful. Second and third degree burns – where the skin blisters and blackens – need urgent medical attention.

Sunburn is always caused by overexposure to the sun's ultra-violet (UV) rays. There are two types – UVA and UVB – and scientists now admit they were wrong to think only the UVB rays were dangerous. Both will damage the skin. UVB rays attack the outer layer while UVA go even deeper to damage the collagen that gives skin its elasticity. Indeed, far from being harmless, the UVA rays are more closely associated with malignant melanoma (cancer of the skin) and premature ageing than UVB.

According to new reports, a combination of **betacarotene** and **vitamin E** supplements can work together in the body to protect against burning. Betacarotenes, the substances that give fruit and plants their bright colours, protect plants against damage from UV light and early research suggests they may do the same for humans. In adult trials, reported in the proceedings of the Society for Experimental Biology and Medicine, twenty-two volunteers were given increasing doses of betacarotenes over twenty-four weeks. Researchers measured their skin's sensitivity to sunlight and found that, as the dose increased, the skin became more protected from sunburn. A second study, published in the *American Journal of Clinical Nutrition*, found that taking vitamin E (500 IU) along with betacarotenes (25mg) for twelve weeks increased the amount of protection even more. In animal studies, it was also shown to protect against skin cancers and premature ageing.

What to do

To prevent sunburn, keep your child covered and out of the intense midday sun. Use a sun protection cream made from the **edelweiss** plant which grows so high it has its own built-in SPF (sun protection factor). Edelweiss sun lotion is a new herbal cream from **Green People** (01444 401444) which comes in two SPF strengths. A 200ml bottle of 15 SPF costs £14.99. The same size bottle of 22 SPF costs £15.99. **Desert Sun** tanning lotion from **Desert Essence** has an SPF of 15 and combines aloe vera with shea butter, vitamin E and betacarotene. 120ml costs £5.95.

If your child has burned, spray the affected areas with **colloidal silver** (see page 297) to promote rapid tissue healing and give 250mg of the **amino acid L-cysteine** which specifically promotes the healing of burns. (This supplement should be taken on an empty stomach.) Optima Healthcare's soothing **aloe vera gel** is 99.9 per cent pure and will not only take the sting out but act as a disinfectant too. It costs £4.99 for 200ml. Keep a **Burt's Bees comfrey ointment** in the first aid kit. It costs just £3.50 from Farmacia (020 7404 8808) and is fantastically healing.

Flower power Australian bush remedy: Mulla Mulla, which helps release stored radiation from the body. Some people report the bizarre reaction of reliving previous experiences of sunburn when they take this remedy for the first time. Thankfully, if this does happen, it will pass within a day or two.

Teen Spots

What's happening?

It's one of life's crueller ironies that 'zits' always hit right at the age when how you look and how attractive you are to the opposite sex matters most. The fact is that the skin is a mirror to the inside of the body, reflecting not only the health of all the other organs but also hormonal changes.

In Chinese medicine, the skin is known as the fourth organ of elimination. The colon, liver and kidneys are the organs responsible for clearing the body of toxins. What happens when they are overburdened with mucus and toxic waste matter is that the skin (and lungs) take over. But this is only one of a number of hidden reasons for getting spots. If you are tackling acne, which is not the same problem, see page 289.

What to do

Constipation is often linked with skin problems so if this is a factor you need to address what is going on with the digestion (see page 251). A high-fat, high-sugar and low-fibre diet will also increase the risk of skin outbreaks so try to cut down consumption of processed foods and give the kids a good quality **probiotic** (see page 95).

Foods that have the worst impact on the skin include cheese, milk, sugar, fried foods, peanut butter and ice cream – in other words, foods that have become pretty much the staple of western-style eating. Try to avoid these foods at home and encourage your teens to start the day with a glass of **fresh carrot juice** with parsley and celery. This will be rich in **vitamin A** and **zinc**, both of which help promote healthy skin. The kids may grumble about the taste, so appeal to their vanity!

The **B vitamins**, all of which work best when taken together, are also crucial for healthy skin and **vitamin E** will help prevent those fats that are stored in the body from having a harmful effect, so give your teen a good quality multivitamin, plus a B complex supplement. Biocare's **Vitasorb Multivitamin** liquid costs £8.25 for 30ml. Mail-order on 0121 433 3727. The same company makes a good quality, lower-dose **B complex** for younger kids who may be having skin problems too: 30 veggie capsules cost £2.70.

Chlorophyll can also help. If you can persuade them to drink it – be warned, it looks and tastes like grass – then a daily shot of **wheatgrass** will also help. I like Xynergy's **Sweet Wheat powder** which costs £19.95 for 15g plus £1.95 p&p. To mail-order call 01730 813642. To make up a juice, dissolve a heaped teaspoon in a glass of water. And if they won't drink it, keep it on standby to make an overnight 'paste' which will help treat a spot that does appear and get rid of it more quickly. (Apply the paste to the spot overnight.)

Keeping the skin clean is important beause clogged pores can cause spots, but harsh and highly alkaline soaps will remove the skin's protective oil and its infection-fighting acidity. If you can afford it, invest in the wonderful **Living Nature** range which, despite being made by a trained chemist, contains no chemicals or preservatives. Instead, herbs are mixed with manuka honey to produce a natural skincare range suited to all ages.

You can even think about making your own skincare oils. Teenage boys may baulk at going to this kind of trouble but the girls in the family (including Mum) will get a great kick out of mixing their own **Ayurvedic beauty oil** and watching it work to keep skin looking healthy. You'll need to raid the store cupboard to mix and then massage equal parts of **sesame, sunflower,**

flaxseed, almond and **olive oils** sparingly into the skin at night. If you don't have time, use **Seven Wonders Miracle Lotion** which includes all these oils plus skin rejuvenating herbs. It costs £9.95 and is available only from Ancient Roots on 020 8421 9877.

If this all sounds like too much trouble, use Napier's ready-made **Green Clay**, a wonderful exfoliant that you make into a face mask to cleanse and soften the skin. It costs £4.10 for 50g and so is not beyond the budget of most teens. To order, call 0131 343 6683.

Flower power Australian bush remedy combo: Five Corners, Billy Goat Plum, Bottlebrush, Fringed Violet and Jacaranda. Designed to promote healthy skin but will also help your teen feel better about the obvious physical signs of their transition through adolescence.

Teething

What's happening?

Teething normally starts at around five to six months. Once the first tooth has pushed through, your baby will get a new one about once a month. The rate and order of emerging teeth varies between babies but the first two through are usually the two middle teeth at the bottom, followed by adjacent teeth and then the two middle teeth on the top gum. The molars, which we use for grinding food, are always the last teeth to appear. Children have twenty baby or milk teeth and teething is usually complete by the age of three. Teething babies will be more restless than usual and more prone to nasal congestion and ear infections (see page 327). They will want to bite on hard objects, will drool and may have trouble sleeping. Sore and inflamed gums, a low-grade temperature and increased irritability are also signs of teething. Adult teeth, which start to nudge through from the age of six or seven, do not cause anything like the same discomfort.

What to do

Babies and younger children respond fantastically well to homeopathy. For the best results, find a practitioner. To find a qualified homeopath in your area, contact the **Society of Homeopaths** on 01604 621400. To find a doctor who is also a qualified homeopath call the **British Homeopathic Association** on 020 7935 2163. If you want an over-the-counter remedy, **Chamomilla** is commonly used for babies whose gums are red, swollen, bleed easily and are very sensitive to the touch. Give a **12x** or **6c** potency on the hour for up to six doses. Babies who have delayed and difficult teething need **Calcarea carbonica**. Give **30x** or **9c** potency, twice a day for up to six doses. You can mail-order homeopathic remedies from Ainsworths (020 7935 5330).

Biting helps to relieve the pressure being exerted on the gum by the emerging tooth so give baby something to bite on. Hard rubber rings are best. For extra relief, keep them in the fridge. The cold temperature will help numb the pain.

To relieve sore gums, dilute one drop of **clove oil** in 1–2 tablespoons of safflower oil, dip your clean forefinger in this mix and gently massage the affected area. Repeat this 2–3 times a day.

Teething toddlers will also find relief from chewing on long, thin and sweet-tasting pieces of **liquorice root**. (Mail-order from Farmacia on 020 7831 0830.) You can also make a soothing paste from powdered liquorice root which you then pat gently onto the sore gum area. You can buy quality herbs and essential oils from Napiers (0131 343 6683).

If teething has caused a facial rash, use Napier's **Infant**

Starflower Cream which includes chamomile, chickweed and borage (£4.95 for 60ml).

Flower power Australian bush remedy combo: Paw Paw, Jacaranda and Sundew. Sundew helps the body cope with pain and is enhanced by the other two remedies in this combination.

Travel Sickness – Sea and Car

What's happening?

Vertigo is the name given to a false sensation of moving or spinning accompanied by nausea and a loss of balance. The most common form is, of course, motion sickness, especially in the back of a moving car or rocking boat. Some kids suffer and others do not. It all depends on the sensitivity of the lining of the inner ear, which communicates with the part of the brain that controls balance and equilibrium.

What to do

Travel sickness is easier to prevent than cure so you need to take steps before the journey starts to minimize the risks. Chinese sailors, for example, would chew on raw **ginger root** to stop sea sickness, and in a study involving some eighty modern naval cadets, researchers found that taking just 1g of powdered ginger before embarkation reduced the symptoms of seasickness – including dizziness – by almost 40 per cent and slashed the frequency of vomiting by over 70 per cent.

You can make a thermos of ginger tea to take on the trip or give the herb in tincture or capsule form. Since the symptoms are likely to recur during travelling, give the first age-appropriate dose an hour before setting off and repeat small, regular doses throughout the journey. If using a tincture, give 10–20 drops, under the tongue. If using capsules, **Solgar's Ginger Root capsules** cost £12.55 for 60. Call 01442 890355 to find local stockists. Boots and other high-street chemists and health stores now sell **Sea Bands** which work well with kids. They put pressure on specific acupuncture points (see Acupressure, page 137) on the wrist to relieve both nausea and vomiting.

Ginkgo biloba, which is reported to boost circulation and thus sharpen the brain, has also been shown to be effective in treating sea and travel sickness in older children. Remember, though, that herbs only work because they can be as potent as prescription drugs. If your child is already taking any kind of medication, check with your doctor before DIY dosing. Remember, too, it can take the body several hours to recover from travel sickness and so your child may still be suffering long after the trip is over.

*****

Five-star Tip

Kids who suffer from motion sickness may be restless and feel that moving around will help. In fact, the opposite is true. Persuade your child to stay seated and put a pillow behind the head to keep it still and maintain the balance of the fluids in the inner ear. In the car, open the window for ventilation and try to distract a younger child with a story or tape.

Flower power Australian bush remedy combo: Dog Rose, Crowea and Paw Paw. Restores internal balance and helps the body recover from the shock of sickness.

Verrucas and Warts

What's happening?

These foot warts are caused by a virus which has invaded the skin, causing the cells to multiply rapidly and form raised lumps. The body cannot kill off the virus and so, instead, walls off these lumps, which are highly contagious. The constant pressure of walking on them then causes them to harden and burrow deeper into the skin which can, eventually, make even walking painful.

What to do

The ancient Greeks valued **oregano** for its potent antiseptic properties and would crown newly weds with it. Today, **oregano oil** is often used to treat a range of skin complaints, including warts (on both feet and hands). The key with this remedy is to ensure you are using the real thing and not, as often happens, cultivated and cheaper marjoram which has been passed off as oregano. Products derived from true oregano are from a plant called *Origanum vulgare* so make sure this is the active ingredient you are using. You can mail-order **Oreganol** from Revital (0800 252875). It costs £22.95 for 13.5ml, so use sparingly. To treat the wart, place a few drops of the oil on a clean, cotton swab and gently dab the affected area. Do this every day until it disappears.

If you are taking a DIY homeopathic approach, the over-the-counter remedy for warts is **Causticum 6c**. You can mail-order your homeopathic remedies from Ainsworths (020 7935 5330): 100 Causticum 6c tablets will cost £5.50 plus £2 p&p.

Children over twelve can take immune-boosting **shiitake mushrooms** which have a powerful antiviral action in the body. These are now widely available in supplement form but the Asian mushroom experts in the UK are Stewart Distribution (01273 703461) who run a mail-order service.

Most children pick up verrucas from swimming pools and school changing rooms. Minimize the risk at the swimming pool by getting them a pair of poolside flip-flops to wear to the water's edge. You can explain the risk to older kids but, in reality, there's not much you can do to protect the younger ones from the health hazards of a communal changing room and floor!

*****

Five-star Tip

Have you heard of the bizarre banana remedy? The healing mucilage found inside banana peel has been shown to help verrucas and other warts disappear. To try this, tape the inside peel of a blackened, over-ripe banana over the verruca or wart, cover this with an elastoplast and leave on overnight. Do this for three nights and, on the fourth, add a few drops of tea tree oil before the banana and tape go on. Maintain this treatment for 2–3 weeks and watch the wart blacken as it dies off.

Flower power Australian bush remedy combo: Five Corners and Billy Goat Plum. Five Corners can help your child feel better about him or herself and Billy Goat Plum is for all skin problems.

Vomiting

What's happening?

Vomiting is much more common in children than adults. Infants will often vomit and regurgitate food, especially in response to overfeeding, but excessive vomiting may be a sign of a problem with the digestive tract, in which case you should seek medical advice. Toddlers and older kids may vomit in response to a food intolerance or allergy, food poisoning, overeating or an infection. If overeating is the cause, the regurgitated food will be undigested and the child will at once feel better for emptying the stomach. Vomiting due to a bacterial or viral infection is usually accompanied by a fever (see page 336). Even a heavy cough or cold can cause vomiting where congested mucus has seeped into the stomach. In this case, the vomit will be a watery mix with mucus.

What to do

Peppermint and **ginger teas** will both help soothe and calm the stomach and maintain fluid levels to prevent dehydration, which is the biggest risk linked with vomiting. This problem is always exacerbated when the vomiting is accompanied by diarrhoea. **Slippery elm** also works to soothe the digestive tract and can be given either as a weak tea or in tincture or crushed tablet form, disguised in herbal teas or fruit juices.

If your child has been vomiting, avoid milk and dairy products until the digestive tract has fully settled. Help it to do this by supplementing the diet with a good quality **probiotic** (see page 95) for several months. Give children over twelve **aloe vera** juice in homemade smoothies to help to settle the digestive system. Avoid solid foods for a day or two. Instead, feed your child soft and nourishing vegetable broths. Bed rest will help the body recover.

The over-the-counter homeopathic remedy that will treat both vomiting and diarrhoea is **Arsenicum Album**. If your child vomits again after being given a glass of water, use **Veratrum Album**. For the best results, though, consult a qualified practitioner (see Homeopathy, page 114).

Flower power Australian bush remedy combo: Bauhinia and Paw Paw. Bauhinia supports the body through the transition from sickness to wellness after vomiting; Paw Paw helps the body cope with internal struggles.

Whooping Cough

What's happening?

Also called pertussis, whooping cough is a bacterial infection caused by the bordetella pertussis bug. Highly infectious, it spreads through the air via coughing, sneezing and even just talking. Most children are vaccinated against this disease (see Vaccines, page 5) at two months, three months, four months and again as part of their preschool booster, which is usually given between the ages of three and five.

The incubation period can be as short as five days and as long as three weeks. The average duration of this debilitating infection is between six and eight weeks. In week one, your child will have what sounds like a normal run-of-the-mill cough which gets worse in week two. From weeks four to six, you will hear intense bouts of coughing that usually end with a long, high-pitched whoop noise which gives the infection its common name. This intense coughing can last as long as two or three minutes, and if at any stage your child appears to have serious trouble breathing, call the doctor or take them to casualty.

During an attack, your child will produce vast amounts of mucus, may start gagging and may even vomit. The face will turn red or purple, he or she may become understandably anxious and one bout of coughing can quickly follow on the heels of another. The final two weeks of the infection are a time of convalescence.

This infection is more serious in babies and the under twos than in older children, whose immune systems are usually stronger, better developed and thus more able to fight it off. In very young kids, ear infections and pneumonia are common complications.

Any child with whooping cough remains contagious for up to three or four weeks after the first cough starts. During this time, you need to keep other children away to prevent the spread of infection.

What to do

Severe cases will require hospitalization where a mechanical ventilator can be used to help the child breathe and where excess mucus may be suctioned from the throat. If you are managing the infection at home, **eliminate all dairy and other mucus-forming foods** including milk, tofu and ice cream. Also **avoid giving your child high-sugar foods** which will only suppress the immune system. Overfeeding can prolong this infection so switch to small, frequent meals and make sure your child **stays hydrated** by taking in plenty of fluids in the form of **fruit juices, frozen homemade popsicles** (see page 108) and, if you can persuade them, **herbal teas**. Also **eliminate fats,** which are even harder to digest when the body is under attack in this way.

A **combined vitamin C supplement with a bioflavonoid** will help support the immune system through this onslaught. I like **Biocare's Vitamin C and Bilberry**. Mail-order on 0121 433 3727 and see page 65 for age-related dosages. **Zinc** is another important nutrient for boosting immunity. Again, check you are giving a safe dose.

Whooping cough can also play havoc with the digestive tract. Support it by giving your child a **probiotic supplement** to replace those good bacteria that help keep us healthy. Again, Biocare make a probiotic powder designed for kids. Call 0121 433 3727 for details.

You can make a tea from **marshmallow root** that will soothe your child's throat and respiratory tract. Make a weak tea (see Herbal Teas, page 106) and give half a cup, three times a day. Buy your herbs from Herbs of Grace (01638 750140). Napiers (0131 343 6683) has a **Marshmallow Compound** designed to ease coughing and clear mucus from the airways. Use it with **Lobelia cough syrup**.

A visit to the homeopath will help clear the vibration of this infection from your child to restore well-being. If you cannot afford a consultation, give **Belladonna 30c** or **9x** in the early stages (one dose, four times a day for the first forty-eight hours) and **Drosera 6c** or **12x** if the whooping cough is dry but accompanied by wheezing. If your child complains of a sore chest when coughing, use **Spongia 12x** or **6c**. Give both these remedies three times a day for up to three days.

Flower power Australian bush remedy combo: Black-eyed Susan, Mountain Devil and Dagger Hakea to help the body cope with the stress of an infection.

Yeast Infections

What's happening?

Candida albicans is a yeast that lives in the upper bowel of almost every man, woman and child. There's no good reason for it to be there but it doesn't do any harm either – until a weakened immune system allows it to multiply out of control. In infants, it can cause a mouth infection or nappy rash, and in teen girls a vaginal infection such as thrush. More common in females than males (the latter get a similar discharge from the penis), it can be swapped between sexual partners and taking the contraceptive pill will always make it worse.

What to do

Mothers who are breastfeeding and who have a history of thrush should cut sugary foods and reduce saturated fats. Cold-pressed and uncooked **olive oil** has been shown to inhibit the action of yeast so this should be used in salad dressings. **Caprylic acid** can also kill yeast but nursing mothers should take no more than one capsule a day. They can also follow the guidelines below to remove any infection from their own bodies and thus prevent transference to the baby.

The damp climate in the UK and underlying nutritional deficiencies – especially **zinc** and the anti-stress **B vitamins** – may play a role in a recurring infection in teens so a good multi-supplement* to correct any deficiency will help, but the biggest culprits are dietary sugars and carbohydrates on which thrush thrives. To clear an infection, you need to starve it so get your daughter to **cut out fermented drinks (including alcohol) and fungi, especially mushrooms.** She should also cut back on **tea, coffee and diet drinks** and aim for **eight glasses of pure water** a day to flush out the bowel.

Several herbs will also help clear an infection. **Garlic** is a potent antifungal agent with a strong antiyeast action. It inhibits the growth of candida and will prevent recurring infections if taken in the long term. Avoid garlic breath by buying odourless capsules which provide 900mg per day of the active ingredient (allicin).

*Make sure any additional mineral and vitamin supplements you are using are yeast-free too.

Health Perception's new **Allimax** is the first garlic supplement to contain 100 per cent of the active ingredient, allicin, thanks to a new technique which stabilizes it: 30 odourless capsules cost £6.99. For local stockists, call 01252 861454.

Aloe vera juice heals a damaged gut lining. The over twelves can drink a quarter of a glass, twice a day, but use a product that is high in mucopolysaccharides, the active ingredient. For infants, dip a finger in the juice and swab the inside of the baby's mouth. Thrush is very common after a course of antibiotics so always replenish the gut's good bacteria by using a high quality and age-appropriate **probiotic** (see page 95).

Nutrition Now's Yeast Defence and Yeast Remedy is a two-pronged attack. First you take a combined probiotic with the antiyeast herb pau d'arco and caprylic acid to clear an existing infection. Then you take a homeopathic yeast remedy designed to prevent reinfection. To mail-order, call Victoria Health on 0800 413596.

*****

Five-star Tip

New to the UK, Biocare's YeastGuard contains an odourless extract of garlic to kill off the candida organism, plus a replacement probiotic of *Lactobacillus acidophilus* which works to keep the vaginal tract healthy. In lab tests, this product killed off 96 per cent of the candida infection within twenty-four hours and scientists were so impressed that clinical trials are now being planned. YeastGuard costs £9.75 for a pack of six pessaries. Call 0121 433 3727 to order and keep this product in the fridge.

Flower power Australian bush remedy combo: Spinifex and Kangaroo Paw. Spinifex promotes internal cleansing and Kangaroo Paw will tackle the infection.

At-a-Glance Guide to Useful Contact Numbers

Herbalism

The **National Institute of Medical Herbalists** is on 01392 426022, or try the **British Herbal Medicine Association** on 01453 751389, whose members have different qualifications.

Homeopathy

To find a doctor who is also a qualified homeopath, call the **British Homeopathic Association** on 020 7935 2163. For other qualified homeopaths, call the **Society of Homeopaths** on 01604 621400.

Naturopathy

The **British Naturopathic Association** on 01458 840072 holds a list of qualified naturopaths who combine nutrition, herbalism and homeopathy in their treatment programmes. Referrals are free. For courses in naturopathy – naturopaths treat illness without using drugs and rely instead on herbs, homeopathy or nutrition – write to the **College of Naturopathic and Complementary Medicine** at 73 Gardenwood Road, East Grinstead, West Sussex RH19 1RX, or call on 01342 410505.

Nutrition

The **British Association of Nutritional Therapists** is on 0870 6061284. You will be charged £2 for a referral list. The **Institute of Optimum Nutrition** in London trains more UK practitioners than anywhere else. Call 020 8877 9993 for a list of graduates and their specialisms. At the **Centre for Nutritional Medicine** in London (020 7907 1660) new clients are seen by a doctor and nutritionist. **NS3UK** (www.ns3.co.uk) takes a special interest in kids' health. Call 01344 360033.

Recommended Reading List

There are specific books recommended in each section. Here are more suggestions for parents who want to dig deeper.

- *The Bowen Technique*, by Julian Baker, Corpus Publishing, Chichester, UK, 2001. Leading practitioner and founder of the European College of Bowen Studies explains how this 'hands-off, hands-on' therapy from Australia, which gets fantastic results with kids, really works.

- *The Clinician's Handbook of Natural Healing*, by Gary Null Ph.D., Kensington Books, New York, 1997. Here's all the proof you'll ever need. The first comprehensive guide to scientific peer reviewed studies of natural supplements and why they work.

- *The Complete Book of Ayurvedic Home Remedies*, by Vasant Lad, Piatkus, London, 1998. User-friendly and comprehensive guide to using the traditional Indian system of healing.

- *The Crazy Makers – How the Food Industry is Destroying our Brains and Harming our Children*, by Carol Simontacchi, Tarcher/Putman, New York, 2000. Controversial, yes, and an absolutely fascinating insight into why we should all be doing more to protect ourselves and our kids.

- *The Encyclopedia of Natural Healing*, by Siegfried Gursche, Alive Books, Blaine, USA, 1997. Probably the heaviest book on my shelf. Provides excellent explanations for a good naturopathic approach, drawing on homeopathy, nutrition and herbalism for the whole family.

- *Fats that Heal, Fats that Kill*, by Udo Erasmus, Alive Books, Canada, fifth edition, 1986. The world expert on fats and health explains how eating the right fats will improve your kids' health and your own.

- *The Fragrant Pharmacy – A Complete Guide to Aromatherapy and Essential Oils*, by Valerie Ann Worwood, Bantam Books, London, 1990. Considered one of *the* bibles for both practitioners and beginners.

- *GM Free – A Shopper's Guide to Genetically Modified Foods*, by Sue Dibb and Dr Tim Lobstein of The Food Commission, Virgin Publishing, London, 1999. You know you don't like it and here's the book that tells you why we don't want GM foods on our shelves.

- *Green Guide – Bright ideas for organic living*, Green Guide Publishing, London (updated every year). To order call 020 7354 2709. A must-have comprehensive guide to UK organic suppliers and services.

- *Health Defence*, by Dr Paul Clayton Ph.D., Accelerated Learning Systems Ltd, Aylesbury, UK, 2001. Adult-orientated (that is, this is not only about kids) and often controversial but the author, who is a scientist, is not afraid to tell it like it is.

- *Herbal Teas – A Guide for Home Use*, by Andrew Chevallier, Amberwood Publishing, London, 1994. A no-frills guide showing how you can benefit from the healing properties of everyday garden herbs from one of the UK's most respected medical herbalists.

- *Homeopathy for Children*, by Gabrielle Pinto and Murray Feldman, the C.W. Daniel Company, revised edition, London, 2000. The next best thing to your own family homeopath, this excellent book shows parents how to make a constitutional diagnosis of their child.

- *Introduction to the Anatomy and Physiology of Children*, by Janet MacGregor, Routledge, London, 2000. A bit technical for general interest but excellent reading if you want to delve deeper into your child's changing body.

- *Menace in the Mouth?*, by Dr Jack Levenson, published by What Doctors Don't Tell You, London, 2000. Read this book before you allow the dentist to put any more amalgam fillings in your child's mouth.

- *PCOS – A Woman's Guide to Dealing with Polycystic Ovary Syndrome*, by Colette Harris with Dr Adam Carey, Thorsons, London, 2000. The definitive (and, to date, only) book on this debilitating hormonal condition which affects up to one in ten females, some as young as sixteen.

- *PDR for Herbal Medicines*, Medical Economics Company, New Jersey, USA, second edition, 2000. Does for herbs what the next book does for supplements, but not for dilettantes. PDR stands for Physician's Desk Reference.

- *PDR for Nutritional Supplements*, Medical Economics Company, New Jersey, USA, first edition 2001. Heavyweight bible if you're very serious about learning more.

- *Prescription Alternatives*, by Earl L. Mindell, Keats, Illinois, USA, second edition. Prolific and authoritative health writer specializing in complementary medicine. Here he explores your alternatives to prescription drugs. Written for adults but informative for the health of the whole family.

- *Principles of Chinese Medicine*, by Angela Hicks, Thorsons, London, 1996. Clear and concise guide to a system of healing that many westerners find confusing.

- *Professional's Handbook of Complementary and Alternative Medicines*, by Charles W. Fetrow and Juan R. Avila, Springhouse, Pennsylvania, USA, 1999. One of the best-thumbed reference books on my desk!

- *The Reflexology Manual*, by Pauline Wills, Healing Arts Press, Vermont, USA, 1995. Excellent illustrative photos leave no room for confusion for anyone wanting to learn enough to practise reflexology at home.

- *The Safe Shopper's Bible – A Consumer's Guide to Nontoxic Household Products, Cosmetics and Food*, by David Steinman and Samuel S. Epstein, Macmillan USA, 1995. A comprehensive guide to what's really in thousands of everyday items on sale – large numbers of which you will want to stop buying.

- *The Shopper's Guide to Organic Food*, by Lynda Brown, Fourth Estate, London, 1998. Everything you need to know about organic food and why you need to switch.

- *Special Diets for Special Kids*, by Lisa Lewis Ph.D., Future Horizons Inc., Arlington, USA, 1998. Very American but brilliant for parents looking for major dietary changes that have been shown to help kids with autism, ADD, ADHD, and other behavioural difficulties.

- *What Really Works – The Insider's Guide to Natural Health*, by Susan Clark, Thorsons, London, 2000. Packed with cutting-edge advice and research for the grown-ups!

Index

chamomilla 379
cheese strings 35, 36
chemicals 4, 34, 35, 38
chi 130, 137, 185
chickpeas (garbanzos) 203–4, 220–1
chicken broth 317, 368, 369
chicken pox 309–11, 353
chicory 204
chilblains, winter 117
children, physical changes 235
Chinese medicine see traditional Chinese
    medicine (TCM)
Chinese restaurant syndrome 341
chips 163
chlorophyll 377
chocolate 249, 299, 333, 347
cholesterol 74, 191, 195, 205, 210, 211,
    213, 263, 266
choline (phosphatidylcholine,
    phosphatidylinositol) 241, 272, 327
chondroitin sulphate 245
Chondromalacia patellae 21
chromium 82–3, 207
chronic fatigue syndrome (CFS) 54–7
chrysanthemum 186
Chunky Chickpea Hummus 220–1
cinnamon 373
    tea 373
citricidal 297
citronella 122, 301
citrus fruits 170, 354
CLA (conjugated lineolic acid) 15–18
clary sage 122
cleavers 368
clinical trials 288
clove oil 379
co-enzyme I 55
co-enzyme Q10 56, 265
co-enzyme R 72
cobalamin 71
cobalt 83
Cocoa-colada 171, 196
cod 223–4
coffea cruda 347
coffee 87, 170, 249, 264, 333
    herbal 87
Cognis 26
cold sores 311–12

colds 139, 147, 191, 204, 210, 267, 275,
    318–19, 328, 336, 340, 371
colic 143, 252, 253, 313–14
collagen 212, 323
colloidal silver 297, 375
colourings, artificial 34, 37
comfrey (knitbone) 304–5, 375
    salve 303
complementary medicine 4, 6
complements 276
compresses 107
conjunctivitis (pinkeye) 334
constipation 104, 105, 117, 139, 148,
    207, 209, 257, 299, 314–16, 340, 341,
    372, 376
constitutional diagnosis 115–16
contraception
    barrier method 283
    pill 127, 205, 362, 363
cookery, for children 161
copper 84, 88, 204, 208, 211, 212, 244
cordyceps 112
coriolus 112, 283
cornmeal 173
cortisol 56
cough syrup, herbal 307
coughs 103, 317–18, 351, 385
Country Life 51–2
cradle cap 321–2
creams, ointments and washes 106–7
crisps, cheese-flavoured 35
Crohn's disease 3, 5, 160
crowea 126, 128, 324, 363, 365, 381
cruciferous vegetables (brassicas) 201
curcumin 35, 37
cuts and scrapes 322–4
cystathionine 264
cystitis 117
cytokines 276

dagger hakea 128, 307, 321, 331, 340,
    368
daidzein 282
dairy foods
    allergies and intolerance 311, 327
    alternatives to 174–5, 249–50, 313
    and cold sore virus 311
    and diarrhoea 325

Hamilton-Miller, Professor Jeremy 97
hand reflexology 145–8
hands-on treatments 130, 136–48
hangover 117
Harris, Colette 364
Haryana Agricultural University, India,
    Department of Foods and Nutrition
    161–2
ha tha yoga 261
hawthorn berry extract 266
hay fever 74, 338–40
Head, Christina 11
headaches 139, 186, 208, 292, 340–2
headlice 342–4
healthy eating, concept of 18–20
heart disease 37, 46, 207
heart problems 263–6
heart mass, ratio to body mass 267
Hebrew University-Hadassah Medical
    School, Jerusalem, Department of
    Virology 320
herbal coffee 87
herbal milk baths 367
herbal pillows 107
herbal remedies 183–7
herbal teas see tea, herbal
herbalists 362
HerbCraft 31
herbs 99–110, 258
    buying 108–9
    cooking with 183
    disguising taste 108
    dosages 101
    homegrown 187–8
    immune-boosting 271
herd immunity 12, 13, 352
herpes 55, 103, 198, 311
hesperidin 297
HIB (haemophilus influenza type B) 7, 28, 33
hibbertia 355
hiccups 139
high-fibre diet 361
highly unsaturated fatty acids (HUFAs)
    23, 326
histamines 51, 73, 114–15, 198, 338
holistic medicine 287–8
holly 349
homeopathic immunotherapy 294–5

homeopathy 11, 114–18, 300, 304, 335,
    346, 354, 370, 379, 382, 387
    and autism 26–7
homocysteine 207, 264
honey 47, 165–6, 339
    see also manuka honey
hormones 277–82
    and autism 26–7
    and cholesterol 264
    and endocrine mechanism 236
    and essential fatty acids 24
    and fatigue 56
    and growth 247
    imbalance 289, 363
    and manganese 212
    and menstrual problems 361–2
    and spinach 207
    and vitamin B6 205
    and vitamin D 75, 264
horsetail 304
5-HTP 51–2
huang chi 31 see also astragalus
Human Nutrition Research Centre,
    Cambridge 159
human papilloma virus (HPV) 112–13,
    125, 283
hummus 220–1
Hunza (people of Kashmir) 202
hydrochloric acid 253
hyperactivity 79, 299
hyperventilation (rapid breathing) 260
hypoglycaemia 179–80
hypothalamus gland 281
hyssop 337

ibuprofen 341
ice-cream, non-dairy 164
Illawarra flame tree 275, 321, 358
immune boosters 111, 195, 288
immune response 276
immune system 7, 11, 31, 69, 105, 211,
    235, 259, 268–76, 306, 328, 338, 344,
    350, 352
immunology 268
impetigo 344–6, 355
indoles 206
infestation (headlice) 343
infusions see tea

INDEX   405